Hands On
DYSPRAXIA

Hands On
DYSPRAXIA

Supporting Children and Young People with Sensory and Motor Learning Challenges

JILL CHRISTMAS

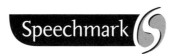

This handbook is dedicated with love and thanks to my husband and family – David, Sam, Charlotte, Kit, Guy, Isabella, Sally – and my close friends, including my friend Eunja Broadie (1942–2007), without whom my life would have been very different.

Thanks also to the Christmas Children's Clinic team – Jenny, Claire and Colleen – and to my editors, including Dr Stephanie Martin, whose positive advice and support kept me on task with this book. A final note of affection to a small black terrier, Benji (1998–2008), a constant companion during the writing of this book.

Published by
Speechmark Publishing Ltd, 70 Alston Drive, Bradwell Abbey, Milton Keynes MK13 9HG, UK
Telephone: +44 (0)1908 326 944 Facsimile: +44 (0)1908 326 960
www.speechmark.net

002-5420/Printed in the United Kingdom/1010

British Library Cataloguing in Publication Data
Christmas, Jill.
    Hands on dyspraxia : supporting children and young people
    with sensory and motor learning challenges.
    1. Apraxia--Patients--Services for. 2. Psychomotor disorders in children.
    I. Title
    362.1'98928552-dc22

ISBN: 978 0 86388 653 9

Contents

Foreword

I first met Jill Christmas when my autistic and dyspraxic daughter
was only 5 years old. Olivia had been unable to walk until she was
22 months and I had taken her to a physiotherapist at Great Ormond
Street Hospital. Once Olivia began walking, the physiotherapist strongly
recommended that she have weekly occupational therapy. I found the
Christmas Children's Clinic and Jill.

I knew nothing about dyspraxia or occupational therapy and found
that there was a whole new language of terminology to learn first.
I might have been quite overwhelmed, but through Jill's kind and
gentle teaching, I found that I was gaining as much from those weekly
sessions as my daughter.

Jill is at the very top of her profession and highly regarded within her
field. What makes her special is her open mind and a willingness to try
new ideas. She has a client list that presents a wide variety of complex
needs and is able to assess each individual on their own merits and,
with careful study, tailor a programme that will give them the
maximum benefit.

Jill offered me understanding and sympathy and loaned me books. Her
approach was fun for Olivia, and through humour and imagination she
was able to persuade Olivia to try new exercises and teach me how to
practise them at home between sessions.

I was extremely lucky to have found Jill. For those who have not found
her equivalent in their area, this wonderful book will be a lifesaver for
a desperate parent and child. It has been written in an uncomplicated
manner and set out in small, bite size steps, suitable for the uninitiated.
We have been crying out for such a book for a long time and I hope it
finds its way into every special needs school and college in the country
and every hospital. Thank you, Jill!

Lady Astor of Hever

Preface

Many of the challenges and issues arising in this handbook may commonly be observed in the general population. Nevertheless, it is when clusters of these challenges arise, affecting a child's everyday function, that the need to recognise the underlying factors and support the child becomes much more relevant – hence this handbook, which can go some way to making sense of the condition of dyspraxia.

Many parents, teachers and allied professionals find themselves in a position where they know that a child is not functioning at their best level within the school or home setting. For example, the child's handwriting skills may not reflect their innate ability, and although it is recognised that there may be underlying issues, adults may feel unable to get to the root of the difficulty in order to support the child appropriately.

There are two main objectives of this handbook:

1   To provide a simple and clear understanding of some of the underlying challenges that children with a dyspraxic profile experience.
2   To provide easy and accessible strategies for support.

The conditions of dyspraxia and developmental co-ordination disorder are often overlapping in many children's and young people's experience. Nevertheless, in this handbook the conditions have been differentiated as in some children they can be observed as separate conditions in their own right – dyspraxia being more sensory based and developmental co-ordination disorder as having a more motor or mechanical base. As the two conditions of dyspraxia and developmental co-ordination disorder are often merged by both professionals and parents, the handbook provides additional sections to explain the associated terminology used and the implications for the children with these conditions.

Each section of this handbook is laid out under three main headings:

WHAT? Definition and meaning of terms used.
SO WHAT? Issues and challenges arising for the child.
NOW WHAT? Practical strategies and ideas to support each area.

It will be noted that there is some overlap in the information provided in the latter two sections throughout the book because the difficulties and strategies are both similar and appropriate across the condition.

This book is far from exhaustive in its information and by its very nature does not cover underlying theory. However, it aims to demystify some of the subtle and less subtle manifestations of dyspraxia and allied sensory motor issues, all of which can undermine a child's ability to function to their best ability in the school setting and in other areas of their life.

Research is continually informing the knowledge, training and clinical experience of clinicians, and I am well aware that some statements and observations found in this practical handbook may not necessarily concur with some current and future research. Nevertheless, these observations are the result of many years' direct or indirect intervention on behalf of approximately two thousand children and offer a practical, 'hands on' perspective.

Some of the information, advice, strategies and exercises may already be familiar to readers in another form or from other sources. It is always difficult to correctly attribute provenance to information shared in a book of this type, but I have tried to ensure that all the information contained within this book is gleaned from personal training and experience, or at least is information for which permission has been given to reproduce. It is hoped that none has been appropriated without reference.

Activities and exercises outlined in this book are advisory only, and responsibility for the safety of the child or children rests with the supervising adult.

Where a child is referred to individually in this book, for simplicity they are referred to as 'he' or 'they'.

This picture, drawn by a young client, appears to reflect some of the confusion and stress that can arise from dyspraxia. Note the drawing of the arms, which may symbolise sensory motor challenges.

Chapter 1

Introduction

I t is with some surprise that I find myself at this stage of my career putting pen to paper to share some of the practical knowledge gained as an occupational therapist working with children and young people in the Christmas Children's Clinic for nearly two decades. My overall postgraduate experience has spanned more than thirty years, and it is as a 'hands on' practitioner that the observations in this book are shared. It is the sort of information that might be shared informally with a teacher or a parent to help them gain a better understanding of what is happening for a child with dyspraxia. As clinicians and practitioners we often have time limitations on our intervention or the opportunity to 'make things happen' for the clients we are involved with at any one time. It seems sensible, therefore, to share some practical experience with those who have little personal time to search out the issues adversely affecting the lives of children with dyspraxia and allied conditions.

In the work at the Christmas Children's Clinic we have had the privilege of working with children and young people who, although highly individual, often present with similar underlying developmental immaturities. It is challenging to observe how these developmental issues impact on the child's higher level functional skills, which are often the first difficulties to be observed – for example, handwriting – while the basis of the problem can start much further back in terms of the child's early development.

If we can understand some of the underlying sensory/motor influences and their impact on function in everyday living, we can then more easily support these children, their carers, teachers and other professionals in facilitating each child's best level of output. It is well known that children and young people with the conditions of dyspraxia and developmental co-ordination disorder are often of average or above average ability in terms of intellectual and cognitive function, and their challenges can be easily missed, leading to frustration and a lower level of functioning.

Despite much research indicating the efficacy or otherwise of therapeutic intervention, resources are often finite in the remedial sense. It seems appropriate, therefore, to provide simple, practical and accessible strategies to assist in effecting a positive change. It is with this in mind that this book has been conceived. Many of the strategies overlap for a range of presenting difficulties and are based on common sense, but they still need to be shared if the child is to be helped.

Everyone who works and/or lives with children and young people has a busy life, and any resource that is to be effective needs to be easily referenced. Therefore, the content of this book is uncomplicated, and ideas can be easily integrated into the flow of a child's 24-hour regime. At the time of writing, I am on a weekly accelerated 'child development' training regime under the watchful eyes of my 4-year-old grandson and 1-year-old granddaughter, who are bringing to life in full technicolour the amazing developmental progression. In this day of evidence-based practice, I believe that 'hands on', anecdotal experience also has a crucial part to play and informs the many theoretical frameworks of reference which are vital in our understanding of the complexity of a developing individual. It is in the role of expert practitioner that this handbook has been undertaken.

Sensory integration has been one of the Christmas Children's Clinic's frames of reference for children with a range of conditions – including dyspraxia, developmental co-ordination disorders, autistic spectrum challenges and sensory integrative dysfunction. The understanding of sensory integrative issues has had a particularly positive effect for many parents whose children have attended the clinic – and also often for older clients with profound sensory motor issues and challenging behaviours. Jean Ayres (2005) and the practitioners who have built upon and expanded her work in sensory integration have provided a wonderful medium for a better understanding of the clinic's clients' needs. It is also appropriate to reference the research, treatment and training undertaken by the Institute for Neuro-Physiological Psychology in Chester under the direction of Peter Blythe and Sally Goddard Blythe (Goddard, 1998; see also INPP under professional organisations on p.153). Their extensive work has provided a much fuller understanding of the impact that underlying neuro-developmental immaturities can have on higher level abilities of children with developmental co-ordination disorders or motor dyspraxia. The Blythes' work has opened up many a practitioner's understanding of the part that poorly inhibited or integrated clusters of reflexes can play in a child with motor learning difficulties. We look forward to seeing continuing research validating the observations and many of the interventions that we as therapists know have changed children's lives for the better, even if it is only understanding something of what is going on in the life of that particular child.

Approximately two thousand children have attended the Christmas Children's Clinic since the early 1990s for occupational therapy assessments, reports and therapy intervention. The emphasis has been on 'making things happen' for these children as well as promoting understanding for parents, teachers, carers and the children themselves of what the issues are and how they might be addressed in a very practical manner. These super children provide the foundation of this book and give validity to what is written. Although it is by no means comprehensive, its aim is to demystify some of the subtle but influential challenges experienced by these children, in order to support them to their best personal level in both the home and school environments.

The role of the occupational therapist working with children and young people with dyspraxia

While occupational therapists are not strictly diagnosticians, they can provide a comprehensive assessment of the child, sometimes contributing to a diagnosis and providing follow-up advice in report format with attendant strategies for the child in their daily life as well as within the school setting. Therapy may also be provided to address the highlighted needs of the child. An occupational therapist may or may not be a specialist in dyspraxia and allied conditions, but if so, is in an excellent position to evaluate the child's strengths and challenges in order to provide understanding and practical support. Close liaison with school staff, feedback from parents and the issues raised by the child themselves all contribute to gaining a comprehensive profile prior to a full assessment. The following assessment tools are some of many which may be utilised by the occupational therapist in order to provide a practical and useful profile of the child with dyspraxia:

- Clinical observations – including the child's engagement with the environment, balance systems, postural strength and stability, ocular (visual) motor skills, body position awareness, co-ordination of the two sides of the body, tactile skills, eye, hand and ear preference, fine motor control, oral motor skills, presence of aberrant reflexes, sensory issues.
- Observations and feedback for activities of daily living or life skills – for example, dressing, knife and fork use, bathing, sleeping and toileting issues.
- Evaluation of physical skills screening using standardised tests, to include large motor movements, manual dexterity, static and moving balance, ball and targeting skills, among others.
- Standardised tests of visual motor integration – testing the combined skills of visual perception and motor recording using the medium of paper (handwriting) or technology.
- Standardised visual perception testing, which includes the more cognitively based skills of visual memory and visual sequential memory.
- Sensory profiling to evaluate the child's level of response to environmental stimuli and the impact it may have on their functioning within the classroom or at home.
- A range of assessment tools to help the child and the parents evaluate the child's performance strengths and challenges.

A child with dyspraxia may or may not have been assessed by one or more other professionals with whom the occupational therapist may liaise, with the parents' permission, to gain a fuller picture of the child's requirements. For example:

1 Paediatrician and/or general practitioner
2 Teacher/SENCo (special needs co-ordinator)/learning support assistant in the UK
3 Speech and language therapist/speech pathologist
4 Physiotherapist
5 Educational psychologist
6 Child and adolescent mental health practitioner
7 Perceptual therapist
8 Optician/optometrist
9 Osteopath
10 Nutritional therapist.

Examples of allied professionals who can support and advise on dyspraxia

The list below is advisory only. It is the responsibility of the child's parents or carers to ensure that the consultants are formally registered health or allied health professionals with experience in the identified area of concern. See the list of professional organisations.

Speech and language therapy may be recommended for:
- Children with oral motor dyspraxia (difficulty with muscular control in forming words, chewing and eating, for example).
- Assisting and advising on auditory processing and organisation of spoken information.
- Children with heightened 'gag' reflexes and allied sensory issues.
- Verbal/speech output and the ability to organise thought processes into the spoken word.

Physiotherapy may be recommended for:
- Assessing the child's postural control, balance and related issues which may be contributing to their dyspraxic challenges.
- General muscle strengthening and building up of core trunk, shoulder and hip stability.
- Inhibition of poorly integrated reflexes: for example, the asymmetrical tonic neck reflex.
- Gait 'walking' patterns.

Osteopathy may be recommended for:
- Postural and musculo-skeletal imbalances in, for example, the head, neck, shoulders, spine and pelvis. These may be as a result of a difficult birth.
- Integration of the sympathetic ('flight or fight') nervous and autonomic systems.
- Ensuring that the body is in balance overall with the interrelating systems: for example, nervous, circulatory and lymphatic systems.

Nutritional therapy may be recommended for:
- Immune system damage which can result in chronic ear infections, asthma, eczema and allied conditions.

- Digestive system imbalances.
- Nutrition and supplements important for brain maturation, in tandem with essential vitamins and minerals to counter toxicity and balance any shortfall, to optimise the child's overall health and integration.

Educational psychology may be recommended for:
- Gaining an overall profile of a child's cognitive and academic strengths and challenges in relation to their schooling and home for reading, spelling, maths, handwriting.
- Advice on emotional and behavioural issues, self-esteem.
- Advice on schooling and placement for a child requiring additional support – including learning support, liaison link between home and school.
- Monitoring and reviewing of the child's progress to help them maximise their academic ability.

The
'integrated' child –
emotional, psychological,
physical, cognitive, spiritual

Gross and fine motor tasks refined

Maturation of personal independence,
behaviours, imagination, cognition, social
and language skills

Functional and physical performance integrating

Eye/hand co-ordination, hearing, attention, information
processing, concentration, visual-motor, receptive, executive
skills maturing

Thinking, organising and 'doing' – ideation, planning, execution

Body control, position awareness and posture control maturing

Sensory systems (hearing, touch, vision, smell, taste) integrating
and fine tuning

Reflex patterns still emerging, maturing and integrating

Body position awareness
Balance
Hearing
Touch
Vision
Smell
Taste

Birth of the baby

Automatic perception of body   Balance (vestibular system)
scheme (proprioception)

Primitive 'baby' reflexes/reactions   Touch (tactile system)

Growth of the baby in the womb

Figure 1   The 'Christmas' Tree: an overview of early sensory motor
development in the child

Chapter 2

Dyspraxia: an overview

The term 'dyspraxia' is commonly used to cover an extensive range of co-ordination disorders. Technically, the term 'developmental co-ordination disorder' (DCD) is the overarching description, with dyspraxia as one profile in this range of conditions. Nevertheless, dyspraxia is still used more generally – as with, for example, the Dyspraxia Foundation. As such, it is recognised by the majority of people as the generic term to explain a range of co-ordination challenges. Other terms used may include:

■ Motor learning difficulty
■ Minimal brain dysfunction
■ Perceptual motor dysfunction
■ Clumsy child syndrome.

These conditions are found in children with normal or above normal intelligence and can present with relatively subtle symptoms, but they often impact on the child's self-esteem and confidence in everyday life. The underlying issues are not easily understood, and they can leave children and adults with a sense of failure and frustration unless they are understood and the right level of support is put in place.

Dyspraxia is often part of an overlapping profile (see Figure 2), and it is not uncommon to have associated challenges with:

■ Attention deficit disorder (ADD)
■ Attention deficit hyperactivity disorder (ADHD)
■ Sensory integrative dysfunction
■ Autistic spectrum disorders
■ Social communication challenges
■ Dyslexia.

Aspects of these conditions are highlighted in this handbook. For the purposes of this book a distinction has been drawn between dyspraxia and a DCD, but with the caveat that the two can commonly overlap. Distinguishing between dyspraxia and a DCD may lead to a clearer understanding of an individual child's difficulties and therefore the subsequent intervention and support.

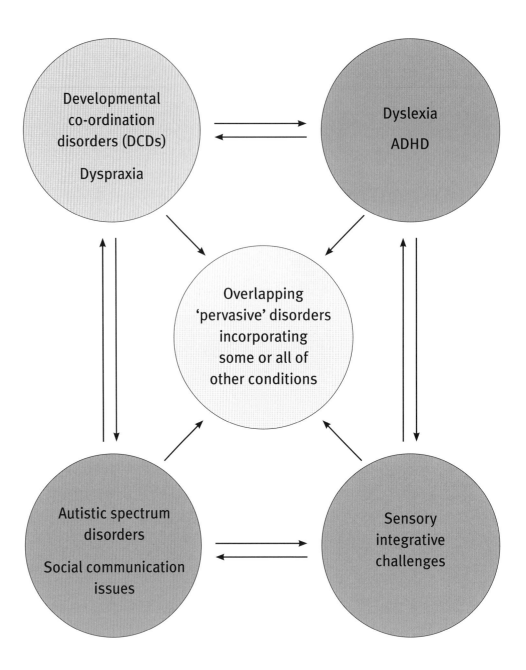

Figure 2 Some conditions may overlap in dyspraxia/DCD

Dyspraxia (sensory motor)

What: definition and meaning

What?

Dyspraxia has been perceived as being due to immaturity of the brain processes resulting in poor organisation, and it can impact on virtually every area of life. It has been suggested that up to one in ten of the population may have dyspraxia or an overlapping DCD. It is also suggested that it is four times more common in boys than girls.

The word dyspraxia is made up of two parts with its basis in Greek:

DYS = difficulty
PRAXIA = planning and automatic organisation of movement
DYSPRAXIA = difficulty in the ideation, planning and organisation of automatic movement.

There are three main components of dyspraxia:

1   **Ideation** – the ability of the brain to think about or conceptualise what the body needs to do (which should become automatic once a skill is learned). The child with dyspraxia may have to cognitively work out which action is needed each time although they have performed the action previously.

2   **Motor planning** – the ability to organise one's body for action without having to think about it. With dyspraxia the child has to consciously think actions through, sometimes at the expense of the task in hand.

3   **Execution** – the ability to respond to input from the environment and make the right movement – in technical terms this is called a 'motor adaptive response' – something that we learn to do from the moment we are born in response to incoming stimuli from around us. Practice refines the movement, and it is then utilised without conscious monitoring.

Dyspraxia may primarily result from challenges in correctly processing sensory information through our different body 'senses' in order to give an appropriate physical response. The following systems are involved:

- Balance (vestibular) systems based in the middle ear
- Body movement and body position awareness feedback (proprioception)
- Auditory (listening and hearing)
- Vision (looking and seeing)
- Tactile (touch sensation)
- Gustatory and olfactory (taste and smell).

All of the above systems need to function at their best level in order for us to organise our body for use and respond appropriately to our environment. With dyspraxia the senses do not always feed back the correct information, and therefore the child lacks 'sensory integration' and their physical (motor) responses are likely to be compromised.

So what: issues and challenges

- The child is of average or above average intelligence.
- The physical milestones of sitting, crawling or walking may all be achieved, but may be slow to emerge and outside the normal time frames expected.
- Muscle tone and strength may be weak, affecting sitting, standing and moving, and the child tires easily as extra effort is required to counter gravity.
- Joints may also be lax or 'hyper-mobile', causing a loss of stability in trunk, limbs and hand control. The child may experience discomfort in back and neck and when writing for extended periods.
- Accident proneness and the tendency to bump into, fall over and knock against objects is common. Objects are knocked over or easily dropped as the child does not always 'register' the force they are using due to poor sensory (touch or body awareness) feedback (see spatial awareness below).
- The child may lack awareness of the position of their arms and legs in space when outside their field of vision (spatial awareness).
- New activities may be difficult to learn and more time is needed to acquire new skills (ideation).
- Articulation and oral (mouth) motor skills may be poor, and the child's speech may be hard to understand; they may also have difficulty chewing and swallowing food. Meals may be a messy business as the child cannot monitor their movement and hand and mouth co-ordination outside their visual field when taking food to the mouth.
- Dressing may be difficult and clothes tend to be untidy, poorly tucked in and disorganised due to a reduced sense of their body scheme and poor registration of touch. Buttons and fasteners are difficult to do up due to impaired manual dexterity and manipulation, and reduced touch and movement feedback.
- The child who does not register touch in the usual manner may overreact to simple touch due to hypersensitivity, or alternatively not register pain or discomfort in the usual manner and appear stoic. (Touch registration may also vary in the same child.)
- Handwriting may be immature and inconsistent in size and form, therefore not reflecting the child's innate intelligence and ability. Free drawing may be poor and again not reflect the child's inherent ability.

◆ The child with dyspraxia can find it difficult to organise themselves and their belongings and forget what they were supposed to be doing.

◆ Short-term memory may be poor, instructions difficult to recall, and the child appear lazy, when in reality they are experiencing difficulty translating instructions into action.

◆ Concentration in class may be compromised with loss of focus, particularly when the child's body position awareness (proprioception) is low. They may need to fidget and move around on their seat to maintain physical alertness.

◆ Social skills may be challenged due to a lack of confidence and self-esteem and resulting awkwardness. The child may be reluctant to engage in anything new, causing social isolation.

◆ Visual perception may be a challenge, although in the author's experience children and young people with dyspraxia often have reasonable visual perception, with some exceptions.

Now what?

Now what: practical strategies and ideas

- Postural support should be provided for extended periods of sitting. Ensure that the desk is at least elbow height, and ideally the surface at a 20 degree angle for school and homework (angled board or file placed appropriately). The chair height should allow feet to be placed firmly on the ground to offer stability and 'sensory' (proprioceptive) feedback.

- Always seat the child facing the focus of the teaching, limiting the necessity to twist and turn; this also allows a 'multi-sensory' approach to teaching – looking, hearing and also observing the teacher's 'body language'.

- Place the child in class where focus can be maintained at the best level – keeping out of the way of main circulation areas assists focus.

- Whole class teaching is ideal, enabling a multi-sensory method of information processing during the lesson and maximum concentration.

- Handwriting difficulties are very common. In class ensure that there is adequate space for forearm support at the desk when writing or typing. Use of textured inbuilt moulded pen grips providing touch feedback and easing of pressure on the pen will assist.

- The child will require strategies in place to assist organisation – see the section on organisation in Chapter 6. Give the child the opportunity to plan and organise belongings ahead of time, and provide a visual timetable where it can be seen easily and replicated at home and school. Give a two-minute warning for any transition to allow closure of the existing task.

- Ensure that the child with poor ideation and planning has good peer support in the playground and in class. Provide positive feedback for effort made as opposed to the end result. Give them personal responsibility for a manageable and regular task which fits in with their personal strength to build their self-esteem.

- Overlearning of motor skills may be required and opportunities for a subtle differentiation in physical education (PE), games and allied activities. 'Splinter' (isolated) skills may be acquired when the child is motivated, but most activities will require extra practice until 'laid down' in the long-term memory part of the brain.

- Ensure that staff are aware that the child may overreact to pushing and nudging if 'touch sensitive'. Place them at the beginning of a queue or where contact is less likely to occur.

- Alternatively, if the child has a reduced sense of touch, check for any injury in contact sports such as football or rugby to ensure safety as they may lack awareness of injury incurred. Also monitor the amount of force a child with dyspraxia uses as they may unwittingly use excessive pressure as a result of reduced sensory feedback.

- Monitor for joint laxity as a child with weaker muscle tone may be more vulnerable to injury and should not be put in a position of heavy weight bearing – as, for example, in rugby – and heavy lifting and handling.

- Advice from a speech and language therapist may be needed to facilitate the child's oral, expressive and eating skills.

- A comprehensive assessment may be sought from an occupational therapist who can advise both the parents and the school on the child's individual sensory and motor needs in order to provide practical strategies and intervention.

Developmental co-ordination disorder/ motor dyspraxia (DCD)

What: definition and meaning

What?

There can be and often is an overlapping profile between dyspraxia and a DCD, and, as noted above, they are often treated as one overarching condition. Nevertheless, throughout this book dyspraxia and developmental co-ordination disorder have been distinguished.

DCD in its purer form may present with a primarily physical profile, as opposed to resulting from sensory issues, and may include:

- Poorly integrated reflexes and postural reactions.
- Immature whole movement patterns adversely affecting gross and fine motor skills.
- A lack of co-ordination and integration of both sides of the body.

So what: issues and challenges

So what?

- The child has normal or above average intelligence.
- Motor milestones may be within average range, but crawling may be missed out or an unusual crawling pattern such as 'commando' or 'bottom shuffling' can occur; walking may be early.
- In school the child may find it difficult to maintain an upright position at the desk despite reasonable muscle tone. They tend to 'slump' over the desk, lean their head onto their arms, or 'head prop' on one hand at the expense of steadying or stabilising their work.
- The child may be uncomfortable sitting in a flexed position at the desk, fidget and experience a loss of concentration. They may have a tendency to sit with legs twisted around chair legs at the desk, prefer to sit on their feet on the chair or alternatively lean back, stretching their arms and legs out in front of them in an effort to feel 'mechanically' comfortable.
- When writing or drawing the child may shift their body to the left or right on the chair, turn their body or rotate their paper when drawing across their body midline, due to poor integration between the two

sides of the body – the lack of bilateral integration hinders the child from working across the midline of their body.

◆ Associated mouth (overflow) movements may be noted when undertaking resisted manual tasks such as cutting and writing.

◆ The above characteristics can indicate retention of the primitive or 'baby' reflexes which cause immature whole movement patterns. These in turn can limit the child's refinement of their arm and hand control (see the sections on symmetrical and asymmetrical tonic neck reflexes in Chapter 7).

◆ The child may hold the pen in an immature grip with the thumb lapped across the shaft of the pen as opposed to a tripod grip with the fingers on the barrel of the pen; in tandem with retained whole arm movement patterns, this can cause fatigue when writing for extended periods. The child may revert to printing letters as they lack the refined intrinsic finger and thumb movements for cursive formation of letters.

◆ The child may be unsure which is the stabilising hand and the leading hand, as they may have an unclear hand dominance and change hands depending on the nature of the activity.

◆ Two-handed activities may be difficult to co-ordinate, including the use of knife and fork, buttons and laces. The child may have a tendency to use whole arm movements with elbows elevated in the air when cutting up food or using scissors.

◆ Some letter reversals may be noted, and dyslexic tendencies are not uncommon in children and young people with an underlying DCD.

◆ The child may have difficulty in keeping their eyes fixed on a moving object in the vertical and horizontal planes, or in looking up to the board and back to their work when copying, and blurring may occur. The child may blink their eyes as an object crosses in front of the midline of their body when asked to visually fix on or track a moving object in the horizontal plane. This may affect smooth eye movement for reading. The child may also complain that their eyes tire although their general vision has been checked and noted as within the norm.

◆ There may be visual perceptual challenges which need to be more formally identified. For example, the child may have difficulty in working both eyes together for binocular vision, and interpreting information such as recognising and matching a shape in a cluster of other shapes. This may be caused by poor 'depth perception' or figure ground recognition.

◆ Swimming may be difficult (the child's face may end up underwater when flexing arms in breast stroke due to the retained linked movements between head and arms). Skipping and reciprocal cross pattern movements can be a problem, again due to a lack of integration of both sides of the body.

◆ Balance may be poor with a resulting reluctance to engage in balance related activities in PE. The child may be fearful of heights.

◆ The child may generally co-ordinate movements well when activities such as throwing and catching are directed to the middle of the body. They may also excel in a variety of preferred sports, but find cross pattern movements challenging as this requires integration of the left and right sides of the body.

Now what: practical strategies and ideas

A DCD may be primarily 'mechanically' or movement based, and a screening assessment and treatment programme are normally required under the direction of an occupational therapist to advise upon and support the identified areas of strengths and challenges. Note also the strategies in the handwriting and visual motor integration sections in Chapter 4 and the bilateral integration section in Chapter 6.

- Allow movement opportunities in the classroom: for example, allow the child to hand out information and provide intermittent short movement breaks to limit 'mechanical discomfort' when sitting for extended periods.

- Provision of an angled board (see resources) or the use of an angled folder to place work on, as this will allow the child to maintain a more upright posture.

- Ensure that the child is sitting facing the focus of the teaching, as turning to and from their desk will adversely affect their handwriting and general motor control.

- Exercises should be advised by an occupational therapist to facilitate integration of both sides of the body and upper and lower body movement patterns, and also to assist reciprocal and cross pattern movements. See additional strategies in the bilateral integration section. Exercises then can be integrated into PE classes for the primary school child.

- Additional exercises are recommended to enhance the child's ability to work and write across their body midline. This will enhance the child's ability to sit at the desk without twisting and turning. Whole movement patterns can be reduced by exercises to help the child isolate shoulder, forearm, wrist and finger/thumb movements under the direction of an occupational therapist.

- A programme of reflex integration exercises may provide positive results – see the sections on the symmetrical and asymmetrical tonic neck reflexes in Chapter 7.

- An evaluation by an occupational therapist for handwriting, visual motor and visual perceptual skills can assist in identifying the primary issues and how to address them.

- Refine hand control with specific exercises to promote a tripod grip and provide handwriting programmes if the child is still at primary stage.

● Enhance functional vision with exercises under the direction of
an optometrist. Advice should be obtainable in the UK under the
National Health Service in most opticians. In addition, advice can be
obtained from the British Association of Behavioural Optometrists
(BABO – see professional organisations). Other countries will have
their own specialists and professionals who can advise on different
aspects of the child's eye functioning.

Oral motor dyspraxia

What: definition and meaning

- Oral motor dyspraxia is primarily a 'motor planning' speech disorder and usually has its basis in an underlying developmental immaturity affecting the child's ability to express words in an orderly and sequential manner. The child may have the ideation of what they want to say but not the ability to 'motor' plan and execute the spoken word effectively.

- Oral motor dyspraxia can also affect the co-ordination of the child's facial, mouth and tongue muscles, which is required in order for them to speak and articulate what they want to say in an intelligible and clear manner.

So what: issues and challenges

- ◆ The child may find it difficult to co-ordinate their mouth and tongue movements, and their resulting speech may be unclear and hard to understand.

- ◆ The child may have had difficulty in copying sounds and early words as a baby and toddler, although they may have the right intonation and speech patterns.

- ◆ The child may have difficulty in the sequencing and organisation of speech and the ability to get the words out in the correct order despite reasonable listening skills and knowing what they wish to say.

- ◆ The younger child may use other forms of communication such as sounds and gestures and may not use words or verbalise speech correctly.

- ◆ Vowels and consonants may be unclear – especially at the beginning and end of words.

- ◆ The child may have indistinct speech and lack confidence in speech production and self-expression. As a result, they may be unwilling to participate vocally in class.

- ◆ As the child with dyspraxia is often of average or above average intelligence, the above issues may engender frustration and reinforce a sense of low self-esteem.

Now what: practical strategies and ideas

- Unless support and practical intervention are undertaken by a speech and language therapist or speech pathologist, the child may continue to struggle throughout their lives with their expressive speech.

- With applied individualised speech and language therapy programmes, many of these children may learn to speak more clearly and appropriately.

- An occupational therapist with knowledge of this area can also support a speech and language programme with the introduction of a range of therapeutic activities, such as blowing and sucking games, which can be integrated into the child's playtime at school and home.

- It is important to encourage the child to participate verbally in class, providing they are given time to organise their thoughts and allowed to speak without pressure.

- Positive feedback for the effort made is vital, and the child's self-esteem and confidence should be supported at all times – the child may appear 'slow' to those around them and thus their skills and abilities underestimated.

- It is particularly important for a child with oral motor dyspraxia to be helped to identify their interests and strengths so that they are able to shine in at least one area. These children may be late developers, and need the opportunity to find different methods of expressing their intelligence and creativity.

- As these children are normally of average or above average intelligence but struggling with speech and usually written output, a full assessment and evaluation of their overall needs can be undertaken by an occupational therapist and/or an educational psychologist to identify their strengths and support their challenges.

Attention deficit hyperactivity disorder

This can be an overlapping condition with dyspraxia (information in this section taken from the Centers for Disease Control and Prevention website – see references). This information is advisory only, and this condition should only be formally diagnosed by a paediatrician or allied specialist, such as an educational psychologist.

For an appropriate diagnosis of attention deficit hyperactivity disorder (ADHD) some of the child's symptoms should be present before they reach the age of 7 and be identifiable in more than one setting. There should be clear evidence of an adverse effect in the child's schoolwork or social settings and their everyday functioning. The indicators of ADHD in a child are listed below.

Inattention

Six or more of the symptoms indicated below need to be present for at least six months, causing disruptive and inappropriate behaviour bearing in mind the child's age.

- The child has difficulty in attending to detail and makes careless mistakes in schoolwork and allied activities.
- They are easily distracted.
- They find it hard to maintain focus on tasks, and their interest jumps around from one play activity to another.
- They do not appear to listen or hear when spoken to directly.
- They do not follow instructions and fail to finish their homework or tasks although they have understood the instructions.
- Organising projects and activities is challenging for the child.
- They dislike and will avoid extended projects in school or homework.
- Equipment such as books, pens or toys is constantly lost or 'misplaced' by the child.
- They can be forgetful in personal care and general life skills.

Hyperactivity

Six or more symptoms of hyperactivity and impulsivity need to be present for at least six months, causing disruptive and inappropriate behaviour bearing in mind the child's age.

- The child often fidgets and fiddles with hands and objects, squirms and shifts in their seat.
- They are often up and down from the seat when expected to sit – for example, during meal times.
- They are often running about when and where it is not appropriate.
- They have difficulty playing with or enjoying fun/leisure activities quietly.
- They are often 'on the go' as though being driven by a motor.
- They may talk excessively.

Impulsivity

- The child regularly blurts out answers before questions have been completed.
- They often have trouble taking turns.
- They interrupt others on a regular basis.

These children may be experiencing heightened stress levels as a result of a poorly integrated Moro or 'startle' reflex. This can keep them in a heightened 'flight, fight or fear' mode – see information on sensory integration (Chapter 3) and the Moro reflex (Chapter 7). Some of the above symptoms may be seen in children with a sensory integrative dysfunction, and a sensory profile should be undertaken by a suitably qualified practitioner.

Autistic spectrum disorders

Children whose challenges fall within the autistic spectrum are very individual, but they may experience what is called a 'Triad of Impairment' (Wing, 2003) which defines their overall condition.

1 Communication challenges
- Speech, communication and language difficulties.
- A lacks of intonation in speech.
- Limited gestures such as pointing.
- Facial expressions and own body language may be minimal, and the child may not be able to pick up these cues from those around them.

2 Socialisation
- Difficulties in engaging with and making social relationships with their peers.
- May have poor social timing and find interaction difficult.
- Lacks empathy and awareness of the emotional and physical needs of others.
- May not have an automatic sense of their own body position in space and stand too close or too far away from others.
- There may be a rejection of or resistance to normal body contact as a result of touch sensitivity, for example, when being greeted or hugged.
- Does not make appropriate eye contact, or eye contact may be very limited.

3 Theory of mind
- Rigidity and lack of flexibility of thought processes.
- Resistance to change, finds transitions from one situation to another difficult.
- Lack of understanding of a situation, particularly if new.
- Obsessional and ritualistic behaviour.
- Preference for engaging in activities, videos and games they feel 'safe' with, and which a younger child would normally engage in.

Children with autism may also have a range of sensory challenges –
for example, a heightened sensitivity to:

■ Touch
■ Sound
■ Vision
■ Smell and taste.

Alternatively, they may have a reduced registration or awareness of pain
or discomfort. They may also have a limited sense of their own body
and limb scheme in space (proprioception). There may be overlapping
dyslexic or dyspraxic tendencies in the child with an autistic spectrum
disorder. Clusters of retained primitive 'baby' reflexes may also be
observed, adversely affecting the child's motor co-ordination (see the
section on reflexes in Chapter 7).

The advice of professionals, including an occupational therapist with
experience in sensory integrative and processing disorders, can provide
a fuller understanding of the issues raised and practical strategies to
support this condition, particularly in relation to schooling.

Dyslexia

The name 'Patrick' was written by a child of 5 or 6 years of age. It demonstrates 'mirror' writing, which may be observed in older children who have visual processing challenges and may be part of the dyslexic profile after the age of 7 or 8.

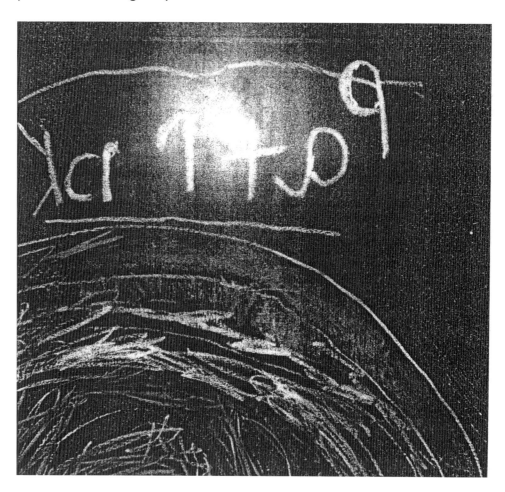

This information is advisory only, and dyslexia or dyslexic tendencies should only be formally diagnosed by a paediatrician, educational psychologist or other suitably trained professional.

This condition can be part of an overlapping profile in tandem with a DCD/motor dyspraxia or stand in its own right depending on the underlying cause. There can be a range of contributory factors: for example, dyslexia may arise from visual processing difficulties or from hearing/auditory challenges. Also, it is not uncommon in children who have immature balance (vestibular) systems, adversely affecting their orientation in space – both for their own body position and for recording information on paper.

Indicators for the child with dyslexia

■ Familial history of reading, handwriting and allied challenges are sometimes seen.

■ 'Jumbled up' or muddled words and phrases.

■ Finds spatial concepts such as left, right, up and down difficult: may reverse letters and numbers and/or tend to lose direction when drawing or writing on paper.

■ May be a very creative thinker and have lots of ideas but has difficulty in recording them.

■ Can be good at concepts with constructional toys but maths may be difficult – for example, with memory sequence or position of numbers and symbols on paper.

■ May like being read to but less keen to read or work with letters and words.

■ Finds rhythm and rhyming difficult – action songs and nursery rhymes are hard to learn in the early years.

■ Difficulty with following a sequence in an activity such as threading beads and recalling what comes next.

■ May have motor co-ordination challenges – for example, a tendency to trip and fall due to a reduced sense of where their limbs are in space, or have poor 'saving' reactions (unable to put their arms out in time to save themselves when falling over).

■ May lack integration of both sides of the body (bilateral integration) and not have a clearly dominant hand, resulting in difficulty working and writing across the body midline, which in turns causes shifting around on the chair.

■ May not have crawled, in part due to retained reflex activity which can 'block' developmental milestones.

Indicators of dyslexia at primary stage

■ Innate and original ideas are hard to get down on paper (although this and other aspects may also be seen in children who are relatively young for their school year).

■ May have an immature 'palmar' (whole hand) grasp when using a pen.

■ Letter and number reversals are still evident after the age of 7 with directional confusion when changing direction on paper as when drawing an angled shape.

■ Time telling and general time management may be difficult.

- Instructions may be difficult to follow.
- Organisation and sequencing an action or activity can be a particular issue.
- May constantly forget and need to be reminded of what has been asked of them.
- May lose equipment, forget books, find planning difficult.
- Large and fine motor skills may be difficult.
- As handwriting output increases, there may be an increasing reluctance to write more than a sentence or phrase when asked to write about a topic.
- Frustration, loss of self-esteem and resulting behavioural issues may be apparent.
- Can be verbally able but work output is poor.

Indicators of dyslexia at secondary stage

- Some of the above issues as in primary school.
- School performance and output does not reflect the child's innate ability.
- Reading and sometimes comprehension may be an issue – may be reluctant to read.
- May have functional eye problems – for example, when copying information from a board they cannot maintain line position when writing, and blurring may occur or double vision.
- Difficulty taking down information when dictated by the teacher. Visual sequential and auditory sequential memory is often poor, with the resulting lack of ability to hold a sequence of information in their working memory.
- Difficulty in setting out work logically and methodically.
- Organisation and completion of projects such as homework – output increases when allowed to use technology, which should be considered as an appropriate strategy with attendant support.

Self-esteem

So what: issues and challenges

So
what?

◆ Children with DCD, including dyspraxia, have average or above average intelligence, but can experience a loss of personal self-esteem for a variety of reasons.

◆ There may be a mismatch between the child's innate intelligence and their reduced functional performance as a result of motor learning challenges.

◆ This may result from an underlying developmental immaturity which has not been identified and is therefore poorly understood by the child and those in daily contact with them.

◆ Avoidance strategies for tasks and activities which the child finds difficult can start to emerge even before they are established in school. They have a sense that they are struggling but do not understand why. As the child is intelligent they 'know' there is something wrong.

◆ A poor sense of self-esteem is also common in children with an overlapping profile of dyspraxia/dyslexia and is compounded by peers, who can be quick to recognise that the child is struggling in written work, games and PE. They can then feel isolated and alone, particularly in a competitive environment.

◆ It is not uncommon for these intelligent children to be placed in low achieving groups in class, as the specific issues may not be recognised or appropriate practical support and strategies provided to optimise their ability.

◆ The child may see themselves as 'stupid', 'useless', state that the work is 'boring', and become oppositional and reluctant to engage in activities that have not previously been successful for them.

Now what?

Now what: practical strategies and ideas

● Additional support and monitoring from the class teacher, providing positive feedback for the effort made by the child, as opposed to purely the end product in schoolwork.

● Should the child continue to struggle and self-esteem be adversely affected, advice should be sought from external agencies to provide understanding and strategies, and to evaluate any underlying sensory motor challenges.

● An occupational therapist with a working knowledge of sensory integration can provide a comprehensive assessment of the child's strengths and challenges, incorporating clinical observations and standardised tests. Strategies and advice can then be integrated into the school day and home life.

● The advice of an educational psychologist can also be extremely valuable to ascertain the child's innate cognitive skills as well as their physical output. Any hidden agendas such as dyslexia or dyslexic tendencies can then be identified to assist the child and their mentors.

● 'Gentle teaching' – initiated by Dan Hobbs in America to support individuals with challenging behaviour – sets out the following prerequisites for success in supporting children and young people with additional needs. Activities and engagement for children with learning difficulties should be:

    (a) Safe

    (b) Fair

    (c) Dignifying to the child

    (d) The 'just right' challenge

    (e) Fun.

● Some differentiation in PE and games may be required, but should be provided in such a way that the child with dyspraxia does not feel set apart.

● Additional practice of specific therapy exercises can be incorporated – particularly for the younger primary age child. The Institute for Neuro-Physiological Psychology can recommend practitioners undertaking this work (see INPP in professional organisations).

● Peer pairing may be of value and also allocating a key member of staff whom the child can specifically refer to for day-to-day issues of organisation, time frames, planning, sequencing and carrying out projects.

- Set functional achievable goals with the child, teacher and parent to enable the child to feel supported and more in control.

- Realistic praise and positive reinforcement will result in a happier and less stressed child; planning ahead and identifying specific issues once a term will also assist.

- There are a considerable number of providers of material to support self-esteem issues (see Speechmark Publishing and Winslow in the resources).

Chapter 3

Sensory integration

Overview

Sensory integration is the ability to take in, process and organise all the information around us, through our different senses, in order to respond and act appropriately within our environment.

- This surrounding sensory information has to be filtered, organised, modulated and integrated appropriately for 'sensory integration' to take place.

- Individuals with a sensory integrative dysfunction and sensory processing difficulties may not be able to process external stimuli in an integrated way, and as a result their responses may not be appropriate to a given situation.

- If these systems are over- or underresponsive, or fluctuate in their functioning, there can be an altered perception in the individual of what is going on not only around them but also within their own body, which may then result in an inappropriate response or reaction.

- For children with sensory integrative dysfunction this can have an adverse effect on everyday life, and their responses may sometimes be seen as emotional or behavioural issues as opposed to what is, in reality, a physiological one. If unrecognised, emotional and behavioural difficulties may arise in the child.

- There are several different senses (sensory systems) through which we process information:
    1   Vestibular (static and moving balance/orientation)
    2   Tactile (touch)
    3   Proprioceptive (body scheme and position awareness)
    4   Visual (looking and seeing)
    5   Auditory (hearing)
    6   Olfactory and gustatory (smell and taste).

Vestibular/balance system (see full description later in chapter)
- If the child's vestibular system is overreactive, they may be very sensitive to movement, avoid unnecessary movement and be reluctant to engage in activities which involve height or very active movement such as climbing. The child may experience car sickness and feel dizzy easily. Their static and moving balance is likely to be

poor, and they may have a poor sense of orientation in space.

■ Alternatively, if the child's vestibular system is underreactive and slow to respond to movement input, the child may be movement seeking and 'on the go' much of the time – swinging, spinning, jumping, running and generally seeking movement in a desire to 'prime' this system and gain the level of stimulation that they need to feel 'integrated' – but usually in a manner over and above the level for their age. The younger child may be very agile and adept at climbing onto any surface they can find!

Touch (see full description later in chapter)

■ A child may register touch in an underreactive way as a result of poor registration through their tactile systems. This can make manipulation and manual dexterity difficult, and the child may also have a reduced sense of their own body scheme, making the organisation and planning of movement difficult. They may be messy eaters as they are unaware of where the food is in their mouths due to reduced sensory awareness. Children with a reduced touch sensitivity may also not be aware when they have hurt themselves, and may appear very stoic in the face of an injury due to a lack of registration of pain or discomfort.

■ Alternatively, many children with sensory integrative dysfunction may have a high level of sensitivity to touch and find handling, touching and the textures of clothes extremely uncomfortable. These children may well overreact to contact with others, resulting in an overt and inappropriate response. They find life in general more threatening and may lose focus or concentration on their schoolwork because of their sensitivity. Hypersensitivity to touch is common in children with autistic spectrum disorders. A child with autism may have a sensory integrative disorder, but a child with sensory integrative dysfunction does not necessarily have autistic tendencies. Children with a heightened awareness of touch may seek contact but on their own terms, and they may 'mouth' and chew things, which is normal in a young child but sometimes inappropriate in an older one.

Body awareness/proprioception (see full description later in chapter)

■ The child with dyspraxia, as mentioned, may have a poor sense of their own body scheme and spatial awareness. There is a tendency to be accident prone, heavy footed (and handed), bump into things, and be unaware of the force they are using in everyday tasks.

Looking and seeing

■ Although a child with dyspraxia may have reasonable vision, the organisation of visual information, its throughput and response may be a little slower – as for visual perceptual tasks. It is also not uncommon to observe difficulties in the child's ability to fix their eyes on a moving object and visually track it in the horizontal or vertical plane. Their eyes may blink or 'jump' at the body midline due to a lack of integration of both sides of the body. Activities such as copying from the board, locating their vision from board to desk, and far and near focus difficulties may adversely affect their schoolwork. Blurring may occur during and following movement. Ball games and allied activities will be difficult as a result. (See the section on vision and eye movement control in Chapter 4.)

Hearing

■ Chronic ear infections may affect the child's ability to hear distinctly, and this in turn will affect speech output. Despite a successful hearing test, very high and low sounds may be missed. The child with dyspraxia may hear but lose focus if in a busy environment due to 'sensory' overload, causing reduced attention and concentration. They may also take longer to process auditory information and require extra time to take information in and respond accordingly.

Taste and smell

■ These senses are very closely linked. Food may not taste very exciting if the child has a blocked nose and sinus problems, resulting in disinterest in eating. Alternatively, many children with sensory integration challenges have a heightened sense of taste and smell, resulting in a refusal to eat many foods. These children may have a strong 'gag' reflex and a tendency to choke and cough up food, especially if sensitive to certain textured and 'lumpy' food.

A multi-sensory approach to learning

Hearing/
listening

Looking/
seeing

Taste/
smell

Saying/
speaking

Touch

Body
movement/
balance

Figure 3 Sensory channels

Learning acquisition – sensory processing

As mentioned, the acquisition of information about ourselves and from the environment around us comes via a whole range of senses. This information has to be received, processed, filtered and organised in order for each individual to give an appropriate motor response to any given input. For some children with a developmental co-ordination disorder or dyspraxia, one or more of these systems may not be functioning at an optimal level. It is therefore vital that other learning methods are incorporated through a multi-sensory approach, especially in the early years, to allow the child to function comfortably and make sense of the information coming in from their environment. From birth babies and children acquire and hone skills which progress from a combination of apparently random, reactive or reflexive involuntary movements to organised, refined and controlled motor output as their systems mature.

Particularly in a primary school situation, desks and tables need to face the focus of teaching to allow both the visual and auditory learning pathways to work together in order to give each child the best chance to consolidate their learning. The child is also able to pick up the teacher's 'body language' and facial expressions, giving them additional learning cues. A twenty-year study at Nottingham Trent University concluded that pupils sitting in rows facing the teacher learn far more than those sitting in groups where some have their backs to the teacher (Hastings & Chantrey Wood, 2002). Professor Nigel Hastings and his colleague, Karen Chantrey Wood, reported that up to 50 per cent of a child's learning can be adversely affected when placed in a group with their back to the teacher, particularly in the case of children who are easily distracted. In their view, although sitting in rows may not necessarily be better than sitting around tables, traditional seating with all the children facing the teacher is far better for most lessons. Some children may be primarily 'visual' rather than 'auditory' learners, so sitting facing the teacher and the focus of teaching is particularly important for them. There is also a requirement for quiet periods to allow consolidation of information.

Every preschool child should be given the maximum opportunity to learn through both child and adult directed activities incorporating movement, exploration and games in the early years. This allows adequate sensory/ motor integration in preparation for school learning. Findings indicate that if a child has not had sufficient opportunity for play experiences, they will be ill-equipped for academic learning, and indeed introducing formal learning from the age of 3 or 4 could be retrogressive for them as they are not developmentally equipped for the demands placed on them. Nevertheless, there are some children with motor learning difficulties who will continue to experience challenges in regard to physical output and require additional practical support and strategies.

The vestibular (balance) system

What: definition and meaning

What?

- The vestibular system is based within the inner ear in the brain and is interdependent with all the other body systems, including the proprioceptive (body awareness in space) and tactile (touch) systems.

- The fluid within the inner ear apparatus (semi-circular canals) contains thousands of tiny hairs, which register and react to different positions of the head, neck and body.

- Messages are then sent to different parts of the body to enable the child to make an 'adaptive' movement response and to interact appropriately with their environment.

- The vestibular system may be oversensitive to movement in some children with dyspraxia, resulting in fear of movement in sport and general physical activities, particularly where balance is integral to the activity.

- Alternatively, the vestibular system may be underreactive, and the child may be constantly movement seeking and 'on the go' in an unconscious effort to stimulate and mature this system.

The vestibular system can influence:

- Posture and level of muscle tone.
- Moving and static (standing) balance skills.
- Functional eye movements and the ability to fix on and follow moving objects in different planes, as well as to move the eyes in a more rapid movement from one place to another.
- Posture and level of muscle tone, which may be low, high or within a normal range.
- Physical and spatial orientation in relation to the environment.
- Integrating both sides of the body together – see the section on bilateral integration in Chapter 6.
- The child's level of focus and ability to attend.

A story is told of a team of astronauts working in space. When temporarily placed in zero gravity with a resulting loss of spatial orientation, they began 'mirror' writing when recording information. When reorientated to gravity, normal writing patterns resumed, indicating that the disruption of the underlying balance systems can impact on writing and recording output. Mirror writing may be observed in very young children and also those with dyslexic tendencies over the age of 7 or 8. This may indicate that immature or damaged balance systems have a role to play in some handwriting challenges. However, this is only one possible underlying contributor to a dyslexic and/or dyspraxic profile; other contributory factors may have a visual or auditory origin, or be a result of motor or general learning difficulties.

So what: issues and challenges

So what?

◆ The vestibular system may be within the norm, but in some children with dyspraxia it is underreactive or overreactive.

◆ If underreactive, the child is likely to be excessively movement seeking, finding it difficult to sit still for extended periods – they need to jump, run, bundle, roll and be generally 'on the go'. As they get older they may seek activities that offer enhanced speed and extreme movement, and the child may appear relatively fearless in their pursuit of movement.

◆ Alternatively, the child with an overreactive or sensitive vestibular system may appear timid, fearful of movement and very wary of anything that challenges their balance mechanisms, even to the extent of experiencing anxiety when going down stairs, and especially on escalators, due to a lack of postural and balance control.

◆ Moving and static (standing) balance may be affected. The child may have difficulty in balancing on one leg, as, for example, when getting dressed. They may have difficulty keeping their balance on PE equipment and be reluctant to engage in play activities involving climbing and walking along kerbs or low walls.

◆ Reading may be adversely affected as the child cannot maintain smooth visual tracking along the line on the page. They may lose their place when looking up at the board and back to their work and/or experience blurring. It therefore takes longer to accommodate their vision when looking from one point to another and to get information down on paper within normal time frames.

◆ The child may have difficulty watching and visually tracking a moving object such as a ball in order to catch it or hit it with a bat.

◆ The child may have rather 'floppy' low muscle tone affecting their exercise tolerance. The ability to maintain an upright posture at the table for extended periods will be compromised, they will tire more easily in class than their peers and may become fidgety.

◆ The child's 'saving' reactions may be weak – that is, the ability to automatically put their arms out in front of them for protection if they fall, causing them to fall more heavily with increased risk of injury.

◆ The child may struggle to organise both themselves and their work in class, and feel as though they are always a 'step behind' their colleagues.

◆ Sequencing of instructions and activities may be difficult, and the child's confidence, attention and concentration can then be affected.

◆ The child may lack the ability to deal with all the extraneous visual and auditory stimuli in class.

◆ The child's ability to co-ordinate both sides of the body for use (bilateral integration) and to work both sides of the body together for reciprocal (cross pattern) movements may be limited.

◆ The child may shift to one side in their chair to avoid working across their body midline when writing across the page, due again to a lack of integration between two sides of the body.

Now what?

Now what: practical strategies and ideas

- Movement opportunities should be provided where possible, prior to schoolwork for the younger child. Linear movement such as swinging and running and also slow rotation movements are soothing, and can provide input to both an underreactive and overreactive vestibular system, enabling the child to attend and focus in their work.

- Provide the child with supportive seating with the desk at elbow height, knees at 90 degrees and feet firmly on the floor for stability.

- An angled board, desk or folder is recommended to maintain good posture and head position.

- Differentiation for recording of information may be required by the teacher. Ensure the child faces the information source in class and is given additional time to record written information. Provide copies of notes as appropriate.

- Ensure the child does not feel overly pressured and that instructions are clearly reinforced in a multi-sensory way (spoken, demonstrated and/or written).

- Allow movement or short respite breaks to ease any discomfort for children with weaker or lower muscle tone and be aware that they may tire more easily.

- Give time for practical organisation of materials.

- Encourage a dominant hand by placing work to the dominant side – this will also stop the child twisting and turning in their seat as a result of any difficulty in working across their body midline.

- Exercises to enhance muscle tone can be advised upon by a physiotherapist or occupational therapist as part of an overall functional assessment.

- A child may have difficulties with visual tracking despite a positive optician's report. Advice should be sought from an optometrist on functional vision (see BABO under professional organisations); this can then be incorporated into the child's school and home setting.

- Give every opportunity to enhance balance at the 'just right' level to maintain confidence and self-esteem. Offer positive feedback for effort made as opposed to the end result where the activity is challenging.

- Plan ahead the night before for suitable books; provide a 'see through' pencil case, ensuring that the contents are maintained in working order.

- Colour code both timetable and subject books; where a laptop is used, provide a copy of an updated timetable as a screen saver or easily accessible document on work/home book.

- Allow some differentiation in PE and games in order to compensate for poor static or dynamic balance while ensuring that the child does not feel set apart from their peers.

- Encourage integrating, cross pattern exercises in PE. Ideally seek exercises from a physiotherapist or occupational therapist trained in sensory integration.

- Allow the child who has identifiable fears to practise activities in their own time and again at the 'just right' level of challenge. Their systems may not be physiologically altered but confidence can be enhanced, resulting in an effective improvement.

The tactile (touch awareness) system

What: definition and meaning

What?

- Our touch system consists of two main parts: one part responds to lighter touch and the other to deep or firm touch pressure. The balance in these two systems helps us to recognise the difference between touch that is helpful or harmful – for example, when handling sharp, hot or cold objects.

- An integrated touch system allows the child to focus their attention and influences body awareness and motor planning. It also allows them to interact with and engage with the environment effectively.

- Many children with dyspraxia can experience a lack of 'balance' in this vital system of touch, and the resulting sensory information they receive can adversely affect their ability to function to their best level – as, for example, in overall co-ordination for fine and large motor skills.

- As the touch system is closely connected with the body awareness and balance systems, strategies are likely to overlap.

So what: issues and challenges

So what?

For children with hypersensitive touch systems the following may occur:

- The child may find contact of any sort unpleasant. They can overreact to nudging, pushing or people standing close to them. They may shrug and move away when anyone attempts to make contact with them, or in the case of a child with extreme touch sensitivity, react in an aggressive manner when contact is made with those around them. (This and allied sensory processing issues (see below) can be common in children with autistic spectrum disorders as well as in those with dyspraxia.)

- The child may find it hard to sit still or focus on what is going on around them, as they have a heightened registration of discomfort from clothes textures and other environmental contact.

- The child may find it difficult to sit comfortably on a hard floor or surface and have trouble getting comfortable and off to sleep at night when bedding is not 'just right'.

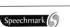

- They may be more sensitive to pain and cry easily as injury and discomfort are registered at a much higher level.
- The child may be intolerant of having hair washed, teeth cleaned or nails cut.
- The child may be more emotional as a result of the above and express anger or anxiety easily. Their systems appear in 'flight or fight' mode, and indeed a poorly integrated Moro reflex may be present which puts the child into a heightened state of awareness, affecting and alerting sensory systems such as vision and hearing (see Chapter 7).
- The child may seek out touch contact by putting objects to their mouth (normal in a very young child) and generally being 'touchy feely', but on their own terms and not always appropriately, as this is a less threatening way of receiving the stimulus their body needs.

For children with an underreactive touch system the following may occur:

- Play activities may be of less interest as touch feedback is poor.
- Tasks requiring manipulation, such as picking up fine objects, doing up buttons and shoelaces, and handwriting, will be difficult due to a lack of sensitivity and feedback in the hands and fingers.
- The child's sense of their own body scheme may be weak. Clothes may be untidy, not tucked in or positioned correctly, not through choice but as a consequence of a general lack of awareness/ feedback.
- The child may not register when they have hurt themselves – for example, if they have rubbed a blister on the back of their heel or cut themselves. They tend to be the 'long suffering' or stoic child who puts up with a lot of discomfort due to the reduced feedback and perception of discomfort through their touch systems.
- The child may not know the force they are using when gripping and handling objects and may break objects easily (also as a result of a lack of proprioceptive (body and limb position) awareness). This can affect motor planning and organisation for activities.

Now what?

Now what: practical strategies and ideas

Strategies for the child with heightened tactile registration:

- Assist the older child to find their own strategies by explaining that they feel touch and pain discomfort more easily than others – particularly if it is unexpected – and therefore need to be aware of this when in crowds, or involved in contact sports and school activities. This will avoid an overreaction on the child's part, as they are more prepared.

- Allow the child additional space where possible in the class setting and around mealtimes – for example, when in a queue.

- When sitting for extended periods on the floor, they may need a small mat or be allowed movement opportunities to ease physical discomfort.

- Ensure that if sensitive to small injuries, these are handled with the minimum of fuss; monitor contact sports/PE to minimise unnecessary problems.

- Ensure where possible that the child is supported in a calm manner; avoid raised voices and minimise noise in a busy situation as this can relieve tension and soothe heightened touch systems.

- At home, ensure that any scratchy clothing labels are removed, use natural materials for clothing where possible, avoid tight belts or buttoning, and provide socks which are heelless.

- Gently rub or massage hands and head at night in the bath, prior to nail cutting and hair washing. Encourage the child to massage gums with a cloth using the index finger before teeth cleaning to ease discomfort.

- Techniques such as brushing the skin and providing therapeutic 'proprioceptive' input can assist in integrating the touch sensitive system – under the direction of an occupational therapist trained in sensory integration. This treatment requires commitment and time on the part of both the parent and the child, but can have successful outcomes in some individuals.

Strategies for the child with poor touch registration and discrimination:

- Prior to a tabletop activity provide movement opportunities for the child to alert the nervous system. Try 'star jumps', running on the spot, stretching out and shaking arms and hands, wriggling fingers.

- Place extra paper under the child's written work to take pressure off the pen. Allow short breaks to ease hand discomfort due to additional pressure in hand and fingers.

- Ensure that games and activities for younger children have a variety of textures and materials to ensure interest and engagement. Use activities with a visual interest as a compensatory mechanism.

- Monitor the child for any injury sustained such as bruising and blisters which may not have been registered by them.

- Where necessary provide adapted clothing such as Velcro instead of laces. Replace existing buttons with textured larger ones for the younger child.

- Provide multi-sensory games such as Twister and the Body Game to integrate body awareness and touch systems.

- Practise action games and rhymes such as Head, Shoulders, Knees and Toes and Simon Says – at a slower rate for younger children – which allow the child to plan and organise their movements.

- It may be necessary to have a full sensory profile undertaken under the remit of an occupational therapist and in tandem with other screening tests in order to evaluate a child's strengths and challenges. The child can then be better supported at school and home with a fuller understanding of their sensory needs.

The proprioceptive (body position awareness) system

What: definition and meaning

What?

This is a sensory system which should automatically inform us of where our body and limb position is in space when outside our field of vision. It is one of the key areas inherent to dyspraxia. Receptors in our joints and muscles should automatically provide this feedback and allow 'motor' planning of movement without any real conscious awareness once skills are acquired.

This sensory system can often be underreactive in children with dyspraxia, resulting in a reduced sense of body and limb position in space in relation to the environment. This can have an adverse impact both on movement and on everyday activities.

Most people can recall a first driving lesson – an exciting but stressful experience. Every action has to be thought about – steering wheel, clutch, brake, accelerator, mirror, handbrake – even before turning the engine on to move forward. Only after careful planning and multi-tasking in the correct sequence can we think about actually driving the car. With practice driving finally becomes automatic, and we undertake a sequence of moves without constant cognitive monitoring.

Children with a reduced sense of their own body scheme and limb position awareness often remain at the stage where every movement has to be cognitively planned, nothing is automatic, and they have to consciously think about their movements, often at the expense of the activity in hand, for example handwriting formation.

Speechmark

So what? So what: issues and challenges

◆ A child with this challenge is experiencing one of the key underlying issues in dyspraxia. Reduced proprioception can result in ongoing difficulties in the planning and organisation of movements, making daily routines much harder and more tiring for them. It can affect all large and fine motor skills, including handwriting.

◆ The child may have difficulty in positioning their body spatially for sitting, standing, getting on and off, over and around or through equipment, or just moving about a room. As a result they may be reluctant to engage in many physical activities.

◆ A child with reduced proprioception may be 'movement seeking' and unable to sit still for long, and they need to move and fidget to remain sufficiently alert in class. This is also common in children with an underreactive vestibular system.

◆ The child may be accident prone with a tendency to trip over their own feet, bump into objects, lack awareness of the force they are using, be heavy handed and footed. When jumping they lack spring and the ability to land lightly.

◆ Physical activity is more tiring for them as they may also have poorer muscle tone and postural strength. A child with low proprioception or kinaesthetic awareness may be perceived as lazy and slow, whereas in reality they are often innately intelligent but lack the motor skills and confidence to reflect this.

◆ The child may take longer to get dressed, dress untidily and be unaware of clothes being inside out and poorly tucked in. The child may be a 'messy' eater and generally poorly organised.

◆ The child may not always register pain and will tolerate discomfort when hurt or injured, in tandem with poor touch registration. They appear stoic and uncomplaining.

◆ Alternatively, some children with reduced body awareness find that their other sensory systems such as touch, hearing and vision are heightened, causing distractibility and loss of focus.

◆ They fidget to 'alert' this underreactive sensory system and find it hard to sit still, or alternatively have loss of focus when sitting for extended periods and 'tune out'.

◆ They may lack awareness of the general force they are using in contact sports, hugging and playing with others. They may break toys and equipment without meaning to and may hurt others unwittingly.

◆ Excessive pressure on their pen, breaking nibs, also causes the child to complain of their hand tiring after writing for a relatively short period as they cannot monitor feedback from the pressure they are exerting; they may keep stopping to shake their writing hand.

◆ Spatial awareness when recording information on paper may be weak. Writing may be messy and poorly co-ordinated, as with general manual dexterity. Laces are often loose due to difficulty in manipulation.

◆ A lack of self-confidence and self-esteem may be observed.

Now what?

Now what: practical strategies and ideas

- Provide the child with warm-up exercises prior to focused work. Gentle push or pull (resisted) activities can alert the proprioceptive system and 'wake' the child up.

- The child should face the focus of teaching.

- Ensure that the child's sitting is symmetrical and well supported, with feet firmly on floor and body correctly positioned to gain feedback through their body.

- Use of a 'Move 'n' Sit' (see Back in Action in the resources) or other design of angled cushion to allow the child 'contained' movement at the desk can be helpful for children who need to fidget to keep alert.

- Allow the child movement opportunities such as handing out books at regular intervals in class.

- Provide the child with an angled board, folder or worktop to assist them to maintain an upright position at the desk and avoid strain on back and shoulders. Laptops should also be angled.

- The teacher should provide extra paper under written work to ease pressure on the hand and pen.

- Allow the child extra time for copying tasks, especially when working from a board.

- Provide pens and pencils with integral grips to ease discomfort and provide tactile (touch) feedback. Advice from an occupational therapist can assist in this and other related areas of function.

- Provide the child with templates, graph paper and visual cues where appropriate to assist spatial presentation on paper.

- Keyboard training with the use of a laptop may be appropriate to ease pressure on the hand when writing, particularly prior to secondary stage, and can then be integrated into the school lessons and ultimately used for tests and examinations.

- Allow the child some differentiation for sports, PE and games in general in order for them to succeed and maintain their confidence and self-esteem.

- Staff should give positive feedback for the effort made by the child as opposed to the end result during activities that are challenging.

Eye and hand skills

Chapter 4

Visual motor integration

There is a strong overlap between the sections on visual motor integration and handwriting as the two areas are interdependent.

What: definition and meaning

What?

- It is the ability to receive, process and interpret visual information (visual perception) and then translate it via a motor act (physically) onto paper with the use of adequate hand and finger control – or with the use of the appropriate technology.
- It is a primary requisite for schooling.
- Visual motor integration requires, among other skills, reasonable eye function, postural stability and upper limb motor control, and visual spatial ability as well as cognitive skills.
- Difficulties integrating visual information with the motor output may be in the visual interpretation of the recorded forms (visual perception), or alternatively in the ability to physically reproduce the perceived information.
- Many children with dyspraxia have a mismatch between their able innate skills and their motor ability – the latter being the main difficulty.

So what: issues and challenges

- Difficulty with handwriting and recording of tasks although verbally able.

- Poor control of pen. Immature fixed pen grip as in a palmar grasp, with the thumb lapped across the pen, or a static as opposed to dynamic 'tripod' (three-fingered grip).

- Whole arm movements may occur, making output more tiring than for the child's peers when recording information due to the lack of refinement of pen control.

- May press too hard on paper or pressure fluctuates on paper.

- The child may tend to 'pen push', which may be due to the retained presence of an asymmetrical tonic neck reflex. An involuntary extension movement of the arm may be elicited by the child turning their head to look at their writing hand. (This movement can be clearly seen in very young babies – see the section on asymmetrical tonic neck reflex in Chapter 7 for further information.)

- When recording information, the child may lean to one side to avoid writing across their body midline due to poor integration of both sides of the body, or alternatively shift their whole body to one side, incurring more effort for them than for their peers.

- The child may not be able to draw intersecting lines past the midline if they lack integration of both sides of the body (bilateral integration), due to the two sides of the body working independently.

- Children who lack integration of both sides of the body (see the bilateral integration section in Chapter 6) may also have difficulty copying from notes at the side of their desk as their eyes fail to work smoothly in the horizontal plane – a midline blink of the eyes may be noted if they are asked to fix on and watch a moving object with their eyes in the horizontal position.

- The child may slump over the desk or head prop on one hand; the distance between hand and eye then becomes too short to sustain consistent eye muscle contraction, which can cause eyestrain (the distance should be a forearm length between eyes and paper).

- The child may not sit correctly on their chair due to a reduced sense of their body position awareness in space, and may need to be reminded to place themselves and the chair in the correct position (see proprioception section in Chapter 3).

- Postural stability at shoulders and trunk and level of muscle tone may be weak, making it hard for the child to maintain an upright position.

◆ Poor representation or orientation of one shape to another (spatial orientation) or ability to maintain line position may be noted.

◆ Loss of orientation when changing direction when drawing angled shapes may be noted (this can indicate dyslexic tendencies if occurring consistently in children above 7 or 8 years of age).

◆ Fidgeting and the inability to sit for extended periods may be noted (possibly due to mechanical discomfort as a result of presence of the symmetrical and/or asymmetrical tonic neck reflex).

◆ Fidgeting may also occur as a result of the need for the child to maintain alertness due to an underreactive body position awareness (proprioceptive) system.

◆ Difficulty may be experienced with copying work, graphics and drawing tasks, use of scissors, building models, apparatus work.

◆ Underlying visual perceptual challenges may be a major part of the child's difficulties.

Now what?

Now what: practical strategies and ideas

- The teacher should ensure that the child faces the focus of the teaching and the interactive board or chalkboard when copying and drawing to minimise the effect of whole body movement.

- A formal check of functional vision – see BABO under professional organistions – is advised to exclude any concerns within this remit.

- Improve pen control by integrating activities such as peg games to build up a pincer grip between index finger and thumb, and to help the child to isolate finger and thumb movements. A dynamic tripod grip should be encouraged.

- An occupational therapist can provide a range of standardised and non-standardised tests to ascertain the main underlying contributors to the child's difficulties.

- Exercises can be provided to work on the child's whole shoulder and arm patterns and integration of both sides of the body under the direction of an occupational therapist (reflex inhibition exercises).

- The child's forearm should be supported on an angled board, folder or desk, allowing the hand to be placed correctly with the wrist slightly extended. This allows the fingers and thumb to fall into a natural pincer grip on the pen, which facilitates cursive writing.

- An angled writing surface will also limit the need for head propping and 'slumping' at the desk and ease back and neck tension.

- The child may need additional lined paper and visual cues to assist the correct spatial start and finish on the paper.

- Where excessive pressure is exerted, allow short breaks to relax the hand; also provide extra paper under their work to absorb pressure.

- Provide pens and pencils with integral rubber grips to ease strain.

- Evaluate the use of a keyboarding scheme from the age of 9, which provides remedial and practical support.

- Place the paper to the side of the child's writing hand at an appropriate angle to ease the requirement to write across the body midline.

- Allow movement breaks for the child who finds sitting for extended periods mechanically uncomfortable.

- Provide templates where free drawing is not essential, and give positive feedback for effort made. Use of IT will be essential in secondary school if the child continues to have difficulties. Ensure that they have formal keyboard training prior to a senior school transition to allow use of a laptop to be integrated into lessons as and when appropriate.

- Limit frustration as much as possible by providing practical and positive verbal encouragement for the child.

Vision and eye movement control

What: definition and meaning

■ It is estimated that approximately 70 to 80 per cent of our knowledge and perception of the world around us is obtained through our vision, and therefore good functioning in this system is vital in normal circumstances.

■ Vision is the ability to take in sensory information through the eyes which is then sent to the brain's visual processing centres to be interpreted.

■ The two eyes need to co-ordinate (work together) automatically and effortlessly with binocular vision in order to obtain a clear image to send to the brain's visual cortex, which processes the information.

■ Some children with motor dyspraxia may have a reasonable optician's report, but when their eye movements are tested they are unable to fix on and visually track or follow a moving object in the horizontal or vertical plane, or easily move their eyes from one position to another. This has particular implications throughout their school day and for general life skills.

■ Links between the eyes, static and moving balance, the touch (tactile) and body position awareness (proprioceptive) systems provide postural stability, visual and motor spatial information, allowing efficient motor control and output.

So what: issues and challenges

◆ Visual stress may result in the child rubbing or screwing up their eyes or covering up one eye to see adequately. They may experience headaches as a result of the eyestrain.

◆ The child may find it difficult to look at the board, particularly if sensitive to bright lighting, and their reaction to a white interactive board should be monitored.

◆ Fidgeting may occur as it is difficult for the child to maintain concentration and focus, with the eye discomfort causing distractibility when working.

◆ Tiredness and loss of concentration are common.

◆ There may be a general avoidance of close work by the child, or alternatively they may lean too close over their work, which can increase strain on the eye muscles.

◆ Abnormal postures may be observed when reading or writing.

◆ Blurring and/or doubling of print may be experienced by the child, particularly when tired at the end of the day.

◆ The child may experience difficulty in keeping their place and/or line when reading unless using their finger or a marker. Reading comprehension or accuracy may be compromised, and the child may develop a dislike of reading due to visual stress.

◆ Copying, either from book to paper or from board to paper, may be hard for them due to limited eye movement control in the vertical and horizontal planes, and due to difficulties moving their eyes from one position to another.

◆ Handwriting difficulties – poor spacing, erratic use of lines – in tandem with fatigue may cause a reluctance to engage in written work.

◆ The child may exhibit poor co-ordination in ball games for catching, throwing and hitting with a bat and in team games due to reduced eye and hand co-ordination and an inability to track a moving ball or object.

◆ General frustration with school work and games due to reduced functioning may occur with a resultant loss of self-esteem for the child.

Now what: practical strategies and ideas

- Ensure that the child not only has an optician's report but also an examination by a behavioural optometrist to check their eye movements (functional vision). (See BABO under professional organisations.) Assessment and treatment should be under the remit of the National Health Service and at established opticians in the UK, and similar resources can be sourced in other countries.

- An assessment by an occupational therapist offering an overview of strengths and challenges is advisable. This should include checking dynamic and static balance, body awareness, and providing standardised tests of visual perception and visual motor integration to assist diagnosis.

- The above advice may also throw up any indicators of a visual dyslexia.

- Ensure the child has balanced and where possible natural lighting to work in. Monitor the effect of the interactive whiteboard on the child, particularly if they have sensory integrative issues (see Chapter 3). It is increasingly common for some children to have a heightened and sometimes adverse response to visual and auditory input.

- Also ensure that the child sits facing the focus of teaching and the board to limit the amount of both eye and body movements when working between desk and board.

- Use an angled board to maximise forearm and upright head position – this will help posture, movement of eyes to the board and back again, and avoid unnecessary fatigue. Alternatively, raise the desk up to at least elbow level to minimise unnecessary visual tracking between one plane and another.

- Provide short movement breaks to minimise and ease visual strain when reading or writing for extended periods.

- Allow some differentiation with printouts – using simple text such as Arial 12 point or ideally 14 point in bold print to minimise strain whenever possible.

- Extra time may be required for recording information – visual cues such as lined or graph paper may be required for writing.

- Allow the child to verbalise information in place of written work where appropriate in school lessons.

- Make sure that the child achieves some personal success in ball games and PE by providing achievable goals; peer pair for extra practice in throwing, catching and bouncing a ball or hitting with a bat. For the younger child a large balloon blown up to three-quarter size provides a valuable throwing and catching activity, as it allows time for them to plan and organise their eye and body movement response.

● Allow the child short breaks when working for extended periods at a computer or laptop. This will minimise any visual stress and consequent strain or overload on the child's sensory systems.

Handwriting

What: definition and meaning

Handwriting is a high level execution skill that brings together a whole range of complex sensory and motor abilities. Despite the increasing technology for recording information in children's lives, written work will still have a vital role to play. The following requirements underpin good handwriting but may present obstacles for those children who have not developed sound underlying sensory motor skills through play and other developmental opportunities. For example:

- Cognitive (mental) idea of what is required, motor planning and the ability to transfer information from the head to the page (execution).

- Adequate muscle tone and balance for postural stability and to maintain a consistent upright sitting position at a desk or work surface.

- The child's innate sense of their own body scheme and position in space and tactile (touch) feedback to inform them how hard they are gripping the pen and pressing on the paper.

- Functional eye movements to allow the child to scan and move their eye gaze from one position to another – for example, between the board and desk – and the ability to adjust their vision in both the horizontal and vertical planes.

- Integration of both sides of the body (bilateral integration) to allow the child to work and write across their body midline without having to twist, turn and adjust their body.

- Co-ordination and use of both hands together – one to write and the other to stabilise the work and make adjustments appropriately during writing.

- Integration/inhibition of the 'baby' or primitive reflexes which, if retained, can cause immature whole body and arm movement patterns in response to the child's head movements.

- Flexibility and isolation of movement between shoulder, arm, wrist and the muscles of the hands and fingers for fluidity of pen control and tool use.

- Smooth muscle control and mature 'dynamic' tripod grip with wrist slightly extended to facilitate cursive writing and to minimise any discomfort in the writing hand.

- Visual motor ability (looking and doing) affecting spatial orientation on paper, left/right, up/down and side to side.

- A good motor 'memory' of letter/number shape formation so cognitive monitoring is unnecessary and writing becomes automatic for the child.

- The 'just right' level of focus and attention for the task.

- Good listening and auditory processing skills.

- The ability to take in information from the environment, and filter and screen out unnecessary stimuli in order to give an appropriate response.

- Sequencing and organisational skills.

So what: issues and challenges

- The child may tire easily, tend to slump over their desk or head prop to maintain an upright position, and find extended writing an unpleasant experience. Frustration, task avoidance and stress may result.

- The child may not position themselves properly on the chair, tending to sit at an awkward angle, and not always know the pressure they are exerting through their hand when writing; their arm, hand and neck may ache.

- Poor feedback from the tactile (touch) and body awareness (proprioceptive) systems can also adversely affect the motor 'memory' of letters, numbers and shapes and automatic recall of how they are formed. The child then has to visually monitor their handwriting, usually at the expense of focusing on the content.

- Copying from the board or transferring information from one surface to another may be difficult, causing errors to be made and the child to fall behind in their work, despite their innate abilities.

- Hand preference may fluctuate if there is an unclear dominance. The child may also twist and turn in their seat or shift their body position as they find it difficult to work and write across their body midline. (This may be caused by a lack of integration of both hemispheres of the brain and is not uncommon in some children with dyslexic tendencies.)

- Mechanical discomfort may be experienced when sitting in a flexed position at the desk, causing fidgeting. The child may feel the need to lean their head on their arms, extend their legs or sit on them to ease their 'mechanical' discomfort, but at the expense of their written work.

- Tremor and/or jerky movements may be observed. (Other conditions may manifest in this manner.) The child may struggle with co-ordinating their finger and hand movements and find manipulation and manual dexterity difficult and frustratingly slow.

- Whole arm movements may be observed in a range of everyday activities but particularly when writing, as the child is unable to isolate individual wrist, hand and finger movements. Recording information incurs much more effort for them than for their peers.

- Poor visual or motor spatial output on paper may be noted, and the child finds it difficult to position information correctly on the page. This difficulty is aggravated when the child has to turn round and then back again to their work in class. When drawing angles or changing direction on paper, for example, they may lose their orientation, resulting in the zigzagging of a shape (also a dyslexic tendency).

◆ The child may be easily distracted and lose focus as screening out background sounds is difficult for them.

◆ Verbal information may be hard to process or organise appropriately for writing information down, due to reduced auditory sequential memory (remembering things in order).

◆ The child may have a good ideation or thinking ability but not be able to organise, sequence and express ideas on paper in an automatic manner.

◆ Verbal skills may nevertheless be competent, and recording output can be considerably improved when a laptop or computer is introduced with the appropriate keyboard training.

Now what?

Now what: practical strategies and ideas

- Allow some movement and stretching opportunities prior to sitting to alert the child's body position awareness. Encourage them to monitor and correct their own sitting position.

- The child's desk should be at or just below elbow height, with knees at 90 degrees with good lumbar support.

- The child should face the focus of teaching to minimise physical moving and shifting.

- Provision of an angled board where necessary to allow correct positioning of upper body, as when the head is bent over, the arms may also flex due to associated involuntary movement patterns, causing physical strain. A 20 degree angle is also recommended for a laptop for the correct ergonomic position to ease strain on the child's back and neck. (See Posturite and others in resources.)

- Release tension in forearms, hands and fingers and also increase awareness of arm position in space by encouraging the child to give their arms a gentle shake or clasp hands and stretch arms up into the air.

- Short built-in breaks should be provided to ease pressure on the writing hand. Provide integral textured pen grips to give feedback to grip.

- Check the child's functional vision with an optometrist to ensure that the muscle control of the eyes is functioning well, also that the writing on the board and their own written work are clear to them when adjusting their focus from one plane to another.

- Refine and improve fine motor co-ordination, finger isolation movement and control for handwriting. An assessment and an exercise programme should be sought from an appropriate therapist to mobilise and strengthen the hand and finger muscles.

- If possible, provide a therapy programme to build postural stability for trunk and shoulder girdle under the direction of a physiotherapist or occupational therapist.

- Activities and games can be integrated into PE and free time to enhance spatial awareness, left and right orientation, symmetrical and cross pattern movements – all aspects which are important for pen to paper activities.

- Visual cues, templates and stencils may be helpful in tandem with additional monitoring by a staff member to ensure success. Lined paper and enlarged graph paper may also assist in spatial challenges. Provide copies of notes to limit unnecessary written output.

- If handwriting becomes a severe challenge and does not reflect the child's innate ability, they may need to acquire and integrate keyboarding skills for schoolwork, particularly in secondary school, one or two years prior to the key examinations.

- A personal laptop may be required, and once the child has achieved a speed of approximately 20 to 25 words a minute, typewriting can be introduced to one or two key lessons with provision of a memory stick or appropriate technology for downloading information, including homework.

- The ability to type will allow the focus to be on expression of ideas rather than the child having to think about letter formation and pen control, assisting ideation.

- Typewriting is a remedial hand activity in its own right.

- Minimise extraneous sounds around the child and ensure some quiet time in class sessions. Avoid positioning near to thoroughfares but ensure they are facing the teacher/board/screen.

Additional tabletop handwriting exercises

The following exercises are designed to improve the range of hand movements and strength. They can be group or individual activities – 10 minute sessions three times weekly.

1 The child (or children) should begin by shaking their hands and arms gently to relax them, ease any tension and alert the body awareness (proprioceptive) system.

2 Place forearms and hands palm down flat on the table with fingers placed together but extended (stretched out). Slowly spread fingers out into a fan shape then bring them back together. Do this at least three times.

3 With palms remaining face down on the table, curl fingers and thumb towards the palm of the hand into a tight fist, hold, then release to straighten – repeat three times.

4 Hands still on table, palms down, tap fingertips on the table:
    (a) Make the sound of a horse walking.
    (b) Make the sound of a horse trotting.
    (c) Make the sound of a horse galloping.
    (d) Relax hands by giving them another gentle shake and rest.

5 Using one hand at a time, place each finger in turn against the pad of the thumb, starting with the index (pointing) finger through to little finger and then back again. The child (or children) then try this with their eyes closed and/or with both hands working together.

6 Place forearms and hands back down onto the table. Keep elbows bent and practise turning hands over and back several times slowly. Ensure that the palms or the back of the hands are flat on the table before turning them back. Initially, this may incur associated arm and shoulder movements. Encourage the child to isolate the forearm and hand movements from the upper arm at the elbow. Practise this five or ten times. Once there is a movement rhythm, increase the speed, then slow down and stop.

7 Try activity 6, alternating the movement, with one palm face down and the other up, practising alternating movements with the object of creating smooth hand and forearm control.

Activities to improve pencil grasp

These exercises are designed for preschool and older children with co-ordination challenges, strengthening pincer grip between fingers and thumb.

Equipment and materials required:
- Short chunky chalks and chalkboard
- Chunky paintbrush
- Range of clothes pegs, shoe box or equivalent
- Real or pretend coins, money box or box with slot
- Beads or dried peas/beans, bottle with narrow neck
- Hollow pasta (which can be threaded and painted, shoelaces with extended tips (taped at the end if necessary to extend tip)
- Jacks or pebbles (washed)
- Old telephone directory or catalogue for tearing up
- Table tennis/ping pong balls
- Dried rice
- Chunky pegs and pegboards, posting games with counters
- Lego®, large size initially, reducing size as child becomes more competent.

1 **Use of chunky chalk for drawing on a board**
- Use a vertical board to elevate the hand and forearm, and allow the fingers and thumb to fall into the correct pincer position around the chalk with the wrist slightly extended when the child is free drawing.
- Helper to draw large shapes and letters on a chalkboard which the child can draw or paint over holding the barrel of a paintbrush in the preferred (dominant) hand. Reinforce the correct formation of letters and numbers, and encourage flowing lines, shapes and rhythm.

2 **Clipping pegs around a box**
- Buy different sized, shaped and coloured pegs.
- Clip the pegs around a shoe box or equivalent, and encourage the child to grip the pegs between finger and thumb using the least resistant pegs first.

■ Practise squeezing and taking off the pegs using thumb and maybe two or three fingers initially, if the child cannot isolate finger and thumb movements.

■ Progress to the child using their thumb and index finger – as their fingers get stronger, use each finger in turn against the pad of the thumb.

■ The child can either do this on their own or take turns with a partner in a variety of games and activities, for example, 'peg dominoes'.

3 Posting coins using a money box or container with a slot in it

■ Post the coins singly through the slot, ensuring the coins are picked up between the pads of the fingertips and thumb.

■ It may be difficult for the child to orientate the position of the coin if they are under 4 years old due to less refined 'whole arm' movement control.

4 Posting beads, dried beans or peas

■ Use a plastic bottle to avoid accidents and closely monitor the beads and peas for safety purposes for children aged 4 and under.

■ The child should hold the bottle with their supporting hand and pick up peas/beans or beads one at a time to post through the top of the bottle.

■ The child picks up the small objects between the thumb and index finger to post, then practises with each individual finger and the thumb, one at a time.

5 Pasta threading

■ Use textured but hollow pasta. Keep in a dry container.

■ Use a shoelace to thread the pasta together, ensuring that the individual pieces are picked up between the end pads of the finger and thumb.

■ Encourage the child to use the same hand consistently by placing the pasta next to the hand the child writes with.

6 Jacks or pebbles (pebbles give a variety of textural feedback) – see therapeutic application below

These exercises are suitable for children aged 6 upwards.

- Practise bouncing a small ball and catching it without picking up the jacks/pebbles initially. Ensure that catching is successful over several attempts before attempting to pick up the jacks/pebbles and catch the ball at the same time.

- Pick up jacks one at a time after bouncing the ball and catching it at the same time. See how many jacks or pebbles the child can pick up in their hand by holding onto the ones in the palm while picking up others.

7 Old telephone directory or catalogue

- Tear out one or two sheets at a time with the 'writing' hand.
- Gather up and crush paper into a ball in one hand at a time.
- Use both hands together to make it into a tight ball.
- Throw the balls into a container or hoop with a consistent hand, again preferably the writing hand.

8 Rolling table tennis/ping pong balls

- Use different coloured balls.
- Line the balls up and place hand palm down; flick each one with the index finger over a marked line half a metre away (ideally on a smooth surface).

9 Sticky/tacky rice

- Place wet palm down on some dried rice in a container.
- Turn hand over with the rice on top of the palm.
- Use fingers and thumb to try to take the rice off the palm of the hand. (There may be some resistance from children with touch sensitivity.)

10 Pegs in pegboards

- Use chunky pegs, picking them up between finger and thumb.
- Make random patterns or copy from an original design. Talk about

left/right, up/down and side to side as the pegs are placed to incorporate spatial awareness.

11 Construction activity

- Work with larger pieces of Lego® or a similar construction toy which offers little resistance and pressure. Progress to smaller pieces that also offer resistance as the child becomes more competent with manipulation.

- Ensure that the child is successful in this activity by supporting where necessary, as they may have difficulty in visualising what they want to make or translating their ideas into action.

Jacks or Fives: an example of a therapeutic application from a traditional game

Jacks or Fives requires:

- Understanding the sequence of the activity
- Motor planning and execution of the physical activity
- Eye and hand co-ordination
- Shoulder, forearm and wrist movement and control
- Grasp and release of hand and fingers at the correct moment
- Finger isolation movement when picking up the jacks
- Timing of the sequence of the task
- Using the right force to bounce the ball appropriately
- Fluency of movement
- An automatic motor adaptive response to the bouncing of the ball.

The activity should be broken down into small achievable steps as with any new activity, and time should be given for each part. For example, allow the child to practise bouncing and catching the ball for several minutes until achieved before attempting to pick up the jacks, one at a time initially, progressing to two, three, four and five at a time.

Scissor skills

What: prerequisites

What?

- Well-maintained safety scissors or adapted scissors (see PETA UK and Taskmaster in resources). Left-handed scissors may be required.

The child requires:
- Reasonable shoulder and trunk stability.
- The ability to co-ordinate both hands together for use: bilateral integration.
- A consistent dominant hand to place the scissors in and a stabilising or supporting hand to hold the paper or card.
- The opportunity to sit at an elbow height table to steady elbows for cutting.
- The ability to isolate finger and thumb movements in order to hold the scissors with the thumb in the upper hole grip and the fingers below prior to cutting.
- Sufficient hand and finger strength and dexterity to manipulate and cut out the shape.
- Reasonable body position feedback from arms and hands.
- Adequate visual perceptual and visual motor skills to identify and then cut round a shape appropriately.

So what: issues and challenges

So what?

- Trunk and shoulder stability may be weak, making it difficult for the child to steady their arms and control the scissors.
- The child may not be able to hold standard scissors due to reduced motor control and limited finger and thumb movements.
- The child may not have the ability to co-ordinate and use both hands together or have a clear hand preference for cutting.
- The child may elevate elbows out to the side (as with the use of a knife and fork), attempting to cut 'in the air' as a result of difficulty in isolating forearm and hand movements, thus limiting control of the scissors and card. (This is sometimes seen in children with a retained asymmetrical tonic neck reflex.)

◆ If the child has reduced or low muscle tone, they may find it difficult to exert sufficient pressure on the scissors or to isolate finger movements.

◆ A reduced sense of arm and hand position in space will make cutting unpredictable and poorly controlled, and pressure may vary on the scissors.

◆ The child may have difficulty with integrating the visual and motor aspects of the tasks and have a poor spatial awareness.

◆ A combination of the above challenges may incur frustration and result in avoidance of cutting and allied tasks.

Now what?

Now what: practical strategies and ideas

- Assess for and provide a choice of safety and/or adapted scissors to evaluate the child's best performance – for example, Taskmaster scissor assessment kit (see resources).

- Allow the child to undertake a simple stretching exercise with hands clasped and arms above the head to 'wake up' their body awareness. Alternatively, ask the child to gently shake and relax their arms and hands.

- The helper should evaluate and break down the activity into small achievable steps.

- The table should be at the child's elbow height with work placed symmetrically in front of the child and their elbows placed on the table to stabilise their work and provide postural stability.

- Ensure that the child is helped to position fingers and thumbs correctly prior to cutting, with the thumb placed through the top hole of the scissors and the elbows stabilised to stop the child lifting them up.

- The child can practise cutting by snipping up plastic straws to achieve the correct cutting action. A collage can be made of different coloured straws for the young child.

- Allow the child to practise with thick card and wider lines initially to ensure success. Start with straight lines, then simple angles and curves, and finally complex shapes to ensure success.

- Allow short breaks and gentle stretching of the hands and fingers if the activity is extended and the child tires.

- Give positive feedback and encouragement for the effort made, even if it is not to the required standard (yet!).

- The advice of an occupational therapist may be required in tandem with the evaluation of other fine motor, visual perceptual and visual motor skills if the child has been struggling with a range of manual tasks, particularly handwriting.

- Exercises for postural strengthening and stability, eye and hand co-ordination and to promote integration of both sides of the body may be necessary, with a referral made to physiotherapist or occupational therapist if there are ongoing concerns for the child's upper limb motor skills.

- Checking of the child's eyesight may be necessary by a local optician, who can be asked to assess functional vision if the child continues to have difficulty with practical desktop tasks.

Visual perception

Chapter 5

What: definition and meaning

What?

(See also the sections on visual motor integration and vision and eye movement control in the previous chapter.)

Visual perception is the ability to take in information from the environment via our eyes. The information is integrated, processed and interpreted by the brain to allow the child to give an appropriate response, as, for example, in reading and writing. If visual processing is weak or fragmented, it is much harder for a child to make sense of the incoming visual information and respond appropriately.

The various aspects of visual perception cannot easily be separated from each other, but for purposes of understanding specific issues a child may experience, they are normally subdivided into the following:

- Visual discrimination: the ability to look at and match a shape with an identical one picked out from a group of other similar shapes.
- Visual spatial perception: the ability to recognise a single shape, in a group of identical shapes, that has a part or the whole of it going in a different direction.
- Visual memory (also has a cognitive component): the ability to hold the memory of a shape for several seconds and then match it with the identical shape within a group of similar shapes.
- Visual sequential memory (also has a cognitive component): the ability to remember progressively longer sequences of shapes for a few seconds and match them with the correct group out of several options.
- Visual figure ground perception: the ability to recognise a shape and then find the same shape hidden in the background of a range of lines and patterns.
- Visual closure: the ability to look at a shape and match it with one of several incomplete shapes which would be identical if completed.
- Visual form constancy: the ability to look at a shape and then find it in a group of other shapes, although it may be larger, smaller, turned around or reversed.

Visual discrimination

Visual discrimination is the ability to look at and match a shape with an identical one picked out from a group of other shapes. Here the shapes and forms remain constant, so it is primarily the recognition and matching of identical shapes.

So what: issues and challenges

◆ A child with difficulty in visual discrimination is likely to struggle across the range of visual perceptual tasks and with most aspects of schoolwork – for example, recognising and interpreting simple or more complex shapes.

◆ The child may have difficulties in both interpreting visual information and/or reproducing it accurately.

◆ The child may need additional support and cues with these tasks despite their innate intelligence.

Now what: practical strategies and ideas

● Ensure that a full optician's evaluation is undertaken between the ages of 5 and 7. Also seek the advice of an optometrist who can check functional eye movement skills – see the previous chapter for symptoms of visual 'stress'.

● An occupational therapy assessment which includes a full visual perceptual evaluation may be required to identify the key areas of challenge for the child. The occupational therapist can advise whether the challenges are primarily with visual perception or with motor output – the latter is usually more common in children with dyspraxia. It may, however, be a combination of both.

● Use a 'multi-sensory' approach of look, see, say, along with handling of shapes and objects, to allow the brain to process information through different senses. If one area is weak another may compensate, using a different pathway in the brain to access learning.

● Allow the child to think and speak about the different qualities of a variety of objects in relation to texture, size and shape. Help them to make up different matching shapes, using games such as Odd One Out and Guess Who.

- Draw a shape with a finger on the child's hand (hidden) or back and ask them to identify it; they then repeat the activity with their partner.
- Play a variety of card games such as Snap with different topic cards, matching 'pairs'; also make use of the resources available in toyshops to address this specific area.

Visual spatial perception

Visual spatial perception is the ability to recognise and match an existing shape with another in a group of similar shapes, that has part or all of it going in a different direction from the rest.

So what: issues and challenges

So
what?

◆ The child with visual spatial dysfunction may appear poorly co-ordinated, disorganised and tend to bump into things due to a reduced sense of where their own body is in relation to the environment and others around them.

◆ The child may find ball games difficult as they have problems judging the distance and speed of the ball travelling through space. They also have difficulty aiming at a target or with any activity which needs a sense of distance, as when hitting a ball in tennis or playing netball.

◆ Fine motor skills may be difficult for the child – for example, doing up shoelaces and playing with Lego®. They may also have difficulty with concepts of left and right and demonstrate poor directional sense both in motor activities and on paper.

◆ Letter formation may be messy due to directional confusion and inconsistent letter size and spacing.

◆ The child may have difficulty in working from left to right on paper in a consistent manner and lose their orientation, or the writing drifts across the page. Other problems may include copying from the board, letter or number recognition and reversals, as in children with dyslexic tendencies.

◆ The child may have difficulty working out underlying spatial orientation of written and drawn work – for example, maths layout, position of numbers and again the orientation on paper.

Now what?

Now what: practical strategies and ideas

- The child should face the board and focus of teaching in class as they may find it hard to transfer information across the two planes from board (vertical) to paper (horizontal) – see also vision and eye movement control in Chapter 4.

- The child's desktop should be as clear as possible with only the materials required for the immediate task to hand. Use of a 'see through' pencil case will assist planning and organisation.

- The child can be helped by copying from information next to them on the desk where appropriate (use Arial 12 to 14 point for clarity).

- The child may need extra time for planning and organisation to enable them to remain calm and minimise stress.

- Provide the child with colour coded folders for different subjects which can be cross-referenced on the visual (laminated) timetable.

- Use 'squared' paper (enlarged for the younger child) for pen and pencil work where possible to provide cues for the orientation of work on paper.

- Provide the child with a multi-sensory approach to spatial concepts using items such as pencils and rulers and games to demonstrate 'in, on, next to, in front of'.

- Use markers from left to right to indicate where the (younger) child should begin and end written work – green for start and red for stop – until it becomes automatic for them. Allow extra time for recording.

- For younger children 'Dot to Dot', tracing, stencils and other fun activities can help directionality and position on paper and facilitate manual dexterity and resultant pen skills.

- Pattern copying using magnets, pegs, 'Connect Four', Lego® and similar activities are useful. Assist the child as required to follow instructions on construction activities and to learn to carry written information from instructions across to the activity (ideation, motor planning and execution).

- Homework could include an activity to enhance spatial and mathematical skills using construction games as a medium. This provides a multi-sensory approach to learning when the child is supported to take an interest and learn new 'adaptive' responses.

Visual memory and visual sequential memory

Visual memory is the ability to hold the memory of a shape for several seconds and then match it with the same shape within a group of similar shapes. Visual sequential memory is the ability to remember progressively longer sequences of shapes for a few seconds and match them with the same group out of several options. Thus, there is a cognitive component to these two aspects of visual perception.

So what?

So what: issues and challenges

◆ The child may have difficulties with reading as well as remembering visual sequences of letter or number shapes.

◆ Taking notes and copying from a board may be difficult for the child as they cannot retain the information in working memory.

◆ The child may not be able to remember and carry over information from one visual activity to another or reproduce symbols and information, which can become a source of frustration and stress.

◆ The child may have difficulty sequencing letters and numbers correctly on the page.

◆ The child may find concentration and focus on a task difficult to sustain.

◆ Planning and organising work may be difficult for the child, as well as remembering work and information learned previously.

◆ Visual memory recall may fluctuate from day to day as with other aspects of dyspraxia, and may lack consistency in general application both at home and in school.

◆ The older child may find they have to keep checking visual information – for example, signs and directions – as visual recall is inconsistent.

■ The child may experience anxiety, run out of time and miss appointments due to organisational and sequencing deficits.

Now what: practical strategies and ideas

- Ensure that the child faces the teacher in order to both hear and observe what they are saying – this allows a multi-sensory method for retaining information and reinforcement for remembering information.
- Reinforce information, especially for homework, in written form – check that the child has written down the correct instructions in their home/school book.
- Allow extra time for copying from the board and general recording, as a child with visual memory challenges may have to check information several times, as well as having to deal with the 'mechanics' of handwriting.
- Provide the younger child with graph paper of different sizes to assist in numbers, letters and shapes being placed in the correct orientation.
- Encourage the whole class to be quieter when engaged in copying work from the board to limit distraction.
- Provide an outline sequential format for planning written projects and a large (12 to 14 point) Arial timetable; keep with their core workbooks and up to date. Work through it with the child at home.

Activities for primary school:

- Use fun perceptual motor activities which encourage the child to remember a sequence of directions – for example, copying or tracing colours and shapes. This may help them to hold visual information in working memory.
- Provide a tray of four to six familiar items. The child looks at them for five to ten seconds; then cover the tray after removing one item at a time and ask the child to recall what is missing from the tray.
- Arrange four or five objects in order, then mix them up and ask the child to place them back in order.
- Draw three or four different shapes, letters or numbers on the board and then erase. Ask the child to draw or say what they saw.
- Muddle comic strip or other sequential activities and ask the child to place them back in order.
- Pegboard games: make up patterns for the child to copy or create a design from existing templates in a game.

Visual figure ground perception

Visual figure ground perception is the ability to draw out important information from other background information.

So what: issues and challenges

◆ The child may find it difficult to screen out unnecessary background stimuli, thus losing focus on the main task, object or symbol.

◆ The child may become easily distracted and taken off task.

◆ When reading the child may lose their place, especially when copying from the board.

◆ The child may struggle to find a place on a map, or in written work, due to all the other background information drawing their attention.

◆ The organisation of the child's work may be poor on paper.

◆ Depth perception may be poor and the child may be accident prone as they misjudge the distance of objects in relation to their background – for example, when reaching for a cup or object. When playing games or in PE, the child may struggle to identify key objects such as the ball from the general background.

Now what: practical strategies and ideas

● See information in the section on visual discrimination above and vision and eye movement control (Chapter 4) for advice with regard to the child's functional vision.

● Minimise clutter around the child's workstation and on the board.

● Simplify presentation of work to be copied and allow additional time for this activity.

● Provide verbal prompts and cues and additional help if the child is struggling.

● Assist with scissor work if the child has difficulty maintaining line position. Provide thicker paper and/or wider, coloured lines for clearer definition to practise cutting.

● Clearly label materials and keep them in a consistent place for ease of access by the child.

Visual closure

Visual closure is the ability to look at a shape, then work out which one of several incomplete shapes would be the same, if fully completed.

So what: issues and challenges

So
what?

- When reading, a child may normally only perceive the partial shape of the letter and the brain then 'fills in' the rest of the letter (conceptualising), thus allowing the child to read more fluently. This is difficult for the child with a poor underlying concept of letter and number shapes, and they need constant multi-sensory reinforcement.

- The child with poor visual closure may find spelling difficult, as it requires the matching up of several component parts to make a whole word.

- When part of a shape is missing or occluded, the child may not be able to recognise the whole shape as their brain is unable to recall a whole shape pattern without all the information.

- Visualising images as a whole may be difficult for the child, and they may not 'recall things' to mind – for example, when trying to picture how get to from one place to another (geographical orientation). Map reading may also be difficult for the older child.

- The child may not be able to match individual parts together from a whole constructional activity – for example, a jigsaw – in order to make up the complete pattern. They cannot visualise the whole or see an overview.

- Calculations for maths and multiplication tables may be difficult.

- Gaining the sense of the 'whole picture' for planning and organisation purposes may be a challenge in the flow of the day at school or at home.

Now what: practical strategies and ideas

- Enlarge the written word when the child is learning to read fluently – stories should be short enough to hold interest. Allow the child to break down new words into the sounds of the letters and reinforce at the end of the session. Give positive feedback for effort made as opposed to purely the end results.

- Provide extra support for spelling and recognition of new and more complex words.

- Allow the child to handle and manipulate shapes to give touch feedback when asked to explain the properties of objects.

- Provide jigsaw puzzles at the level where a child is successful, which may not always match their chronological age, allowing time when there is a peer or adult around to direct the child's focus and interest.

- Cut up simple pictures, ideally of a subject that the child has a particular interest in. The child can then arrange them and glue them back together.

- Present a selection of enlarged incomplete patterns or shapes which the child can trace with their finger and describe what is missing.

- The teacher partially covers a picture and asks the child to describe the whole picture in their own words. Also draw half a picture on a folded piece of paper and then ask the child to draw the other half.

- 'Dot to Dot' using pictures with either numbers or letters – the teacher asks the child to guess what the picture will be at some point before completion.

- Help the child to construct three-dimensional models from Lego® or similar construction activities, encouraging them to describe what they are planning.

- Ask the child to fill in squares, triangles, diamonds and other more complex and incomplete shapes.

- The teacher provides stencil patterns (including letter and number patterns) for the child to fill in freehand.

- See the resources for Ann Arbor Publishers and Happy Puzzle Company.

Visual form constancy

Visual form constancy is the ability to look at a shape and then recognise it in a group of other shapes, although it may be larger, smaller, turned around or reversed.

So what: issues and challenges

So what?

◆ The child may struggle to interpret written information on a board – copying may be difficult, especially when rapid changes of information are made.

◆ The teachers' varying styles of handwriting may present problems due to different sizing and change in basic letter formation, particularily with cursive writing.

◆ The child may find sorting and understanding the properties of objects, shapes and symbols difficult.

◆ Altering of shapes and forms or putting them in different positions may be difficult for the child and cause them confusion, particularly when asked to draw them or describe their properties.

◆ The child may find construction activities hard – for example, using two-dimensional information and then translating it into a three-dimensional construction activity.

Now what: practical strategies and ideas

- The teacher should help to minimise clutter around the child's working area and on the board.

- The teacher should ensure consistency with written work for the child to copy; when printing information out, where possible use a consistent typeface (such as Arial 12 or 14 point).

- Alert other teaching staff to the fact that the child is likely to recognise the printed word more easily than different methods of cursive writing.

- Give additional support to the child in design and technology activities.

- Use the many resources in children's books to match and link shapes that are larger or smaller or in a different position.

- Think of a shape – for example, a square, circle or triangle – and ask the child to find similar shapes in the room around them. Match visual shapes with actual shapes that the child explores with their hands.

- The teacher turns shapes around and puts them in different positions and sees if the child can recognise them – overlap them with other shapes for increased difficulty.

- The child is asked to identify which is the larger, smaller, thicker, thinner, etc between a pair of objects. Start at the level at which they are successful and then make the differences more subtle.

- The teacher writes the same word in many styles, colours and prints, together with a range of other words. The child identifies and underlines the one word.

- The teacher encourages the child to match two-dimensional shapes on paper with three-dimensional objects using different perceptual shapes and puzzles appropriate to their functional level.

- The teacher provides a clearly printed sheet of writing and asks the child to pick out lower and upper case letters.

- Provide computer activities which focus on discrimination of different shapes and symbols. Ask the child to trace over squares, circles and triangles, and then copy them onto a chalkboard (for the younger child).

- The child strings or lays out beads or buttons of one shape that vary in size or colour. The child also copies shapes on a pegboard from varying design layouts.

- Provide the child with the 'just right' level of support and motivation to engage in all the activities for visual perception and make it fun, especially for the younger child!

Additional visual perceptual activities for the younger child

- Allow the child to trace simple shapes from a book and cut them out.
- Provide sorting games using objects of different sizes, colour, shape and texture.
- Encourage 'I Spy' games for younger children on walks and around the house, picking out particular objects or shapes from the background.
- Help the child to pick out different leaf shapes on a nature walk, or recognise different grasses and sedges (use of 'I Spy' books).
- Books such as 'Where's Wally' are fun ways to isolate a shape from the background.
- Provide games such as bead threading, making collages and jigsaw puzzles, but with a shared involvement and at the right 'functional' level to maintain the child's interest.

Jigsaw puzzle – a simple activity to enhance visual perception requiring:
- Visual discrimination – recognising the relevant parts.
- Form constancy – seeing and recognising the shapes in different positions.
- Figure ground perception – drawing out the relevant visual information from a background of information.
- Spatial ability – recognising the orientation of one shape to another.
- Visual closure – recognising the whole shape when still incomplete.
- Sequential memory – holding information in working memory when looking around for the relevant piece(s).
- Fine motor manipulation and manual dexterity including good pincer grip between the finger and thumb.
- Light touch control.
- Patience and ability to stay on task.
- Concentration and attention.

Ensure that the jigsaw puzzle is at the 'just right' challenge level for the individual child and that someone is with them to encourage their interest.

Chapter 6

Bilateral integration: working both sides of the body together

This picture was automatically drawn by a child with average intelligence during an assessment, and appears to reflect an innate but unconscious lack of integration between the two sides of their body.

Bilateral integration: an overview

What: definition and meaning

This is the ability to co-ordinate and work both sides of the body together at the same time for use in everyday activities. It requires the bundle of fibres (*corpus callosum*) in the brain to mature completely in order to fully connect the two sides (hemispheres) of the brain within the first five to seven years of life. The *corpus callosum* has the job of facilitating or inhibiting all the information passed between the two sides of the brain. Where the connections between both sides of the brain are poor, one side of the body can appear to work almost independently from the other. This makes it difficult for a child to integrate the two sides of the body together for all areas of life.

So what: issues and challenges

◆ The child may not have a consistent right- or left-sided hand, foot, ear or eye preference when picking up a pen, kicking a ball, using a phone or looking through a telescope or camera lens.

◆ The child may start to write or draw across the paper to their body midline, but then pass the pencil to the other hand to finish their work across the page (this is often noted in preschool children before integration is complete).

◆ Some children cannot physically write or work across their body midline. As a result, the child may twist or rotate their body or shift to one side on their chair (see additional information on the asymmetrical tonic neck reflex in the next chapter).

◆ In tests of manual dexterity, the child may have equally able hands in performing fine motor tasks as opposed to one more dextrous hand, but cannot fully refine one side for manual tasks such as handwriting.

◆ When writing, the child may 'forget' that they have two hands and neglect the supporting or stabilising arm, leaving it down by their side.

◆ The child may find it difficult to orientate one hand to another and be unsure which hand should 'lead' when, for example, tying a knot, using a knife and fork, or doing up shoelaces and buttons.

◆ Reduced co-ordination may be observed for reciprocal (cross pattern) movements such as climbing and skipping and riding a bicycle. The child may run in an ungainly manner, and also have difficulty in co-ordinating their upper body with the lower body – particularly in swimming and allied sports.

◆ An involuntary 'blink' may be observed at the midline of the body when the child is visually tracking a moving object with their eyes in the horizontal plane.

◆ Where there is no clear eye dominance, reading and general processing of visual information may be difficult. When the child tries to look through a telescope, for example, they may be unsure which eye to use. (This can also be due to a reduced sense of their body scheme – see the section on proprioception in Chapter 3.)

Now what?

Now what: practical strategies and ideas

- In class the teacher or assistant can prompt the child to place their helping hand on the work surface within their visual field to stabilise the paper when working. Prompts can be verbal or visual, but regular reminders are important to encourage the child to involve both hands for everyday tasks.

- Encourage a consistent writing and leading hand by placing materials on the dominant side. Remind the child to stabilise their work with the non-dominant hand.

- If the child has a clear one-sided dominance (laterality) but finds it difficult to work across the body midline, their work can also be placed on the dominant side to avoid any compensatory twisting and turning.

- An occupational therapist can provide an overall assessment to assist in identifying which would be the preferred hand if this remains unclear in the primary school child. Advice can also be provided on appropriate therapy.

- Encourage the child to use both sides of their body together in a range of symmetrical activities such as jumping with both feet together, hand clapping activities, skipping exercises, holding onto a baton with both hands to hit a balloon backwards and forwards, as a precursor to working with reciprocal cross pattern movements.

- Opportunities for extra time to practise functional skills such as the use of a knife and fork and managing buttons and laces should be integrated into the child's day so that they are not put under pressure at key times.

- Bilateral integration challenges are likely to affect the child's functional eye skills. While many children may have had a successful optician's test, the functional movements of their eyes may not have been tested. The advice of an optometrist should be sought as this can make a considerable difference to the child's function in school. See BABO under professional organisations.

Organisational and sequencing skills

What: definition and meaning

What?

This area commonly presents a considerable challenge to some children with dyspraxia. The abilities to organise and sequence activities are interdependent and require the child to have clear ideation, planning and executive (output) abilities for everyday tasks.

Sensory motor integration as a foundation to organisation and sequencing abilities involves the following:

- In a child's early years there is considerable expansion of all the neural circuitry and connections in the brain.
- As the child grows, many of these connections are refined or 'pruned', allowing the remaining connections to mature and become 'hard wired' or more fully laid down.
- The child's sensory systems of vision, hearing, smell, taste, sense of touch, body awareness and balance need to become fully integrated in order for the child to function and access the higher level skills which include organisation and sequencing.

So what: issues and challenges

So what?

- In some children there will be an underlying impairment of both sensory and motor organisation, making it difficult for them to respond appropriately to the demands placed on them both at home and at school.
- The child may not be able to think and therefore plan in a logical sequence, affecting their ability to get their inherently good ideas down on paper. They may have a good ideation of what they want to say or write, but planning and/or execution of the activity is compromised.
- The child's work may be messy and untidy with poor spatial presentation, as they have to battle with reduced manual dexterity and manipulation for writing and drawing, as well as coping with their organisational challenges.

◆ It may be hard for the child to prioritise thoughts, and they are easily taken off task and distracted from the activity in hand. Holding information in working memory in an orderly sequence may be a component of this: the child may appear forgetful and generally disorganised.

◆ The child may struggle to plan ahead in everyday activities and have difficulty organising themselves and their belongings.

◆ If the child is given two or three instructions, the first may be successful but the others 'forgotten', and the child can easily become sidetracked onto another activity.

◆ Auditory sequential memory and/or visual sequential memory may be difficult for the child, as well as working through a sequence of tasks.

◆ The child may also miss the relevant point in what is being asked of them unless the question or request is directed specifically to them and then repeated.

◆ Timing may be poor in responding to requests, and the child may appear inattentive and distracted.

◆ The child is likely to leave equipment and materials behind, or take longer to organise their school belongings, when others are ready to attend to the next step.

◆ There may be a degree of generalised anxiety and frustration as it is hard for the child and others around them to understand why everyday tasks take so long and why the child always seems to be one step behind others.

Now what?

Now what: practical strategies and ideas

- Ideally, therapeutic advice and activities should be provided for children at primary school age, in tandem with advice from an occupational therapist experienced in sensory integration in order to address any underlying sensory and motor developmental immaturities.

- There is likely to be a 'mismatch' between the child's innate intelligence and their reduced performance. Provide positive feedback for effort shown in school and home activities as self-esteem may be low, causing frustration and anger. The child needs to be supported positively to minimise the impact poor organisational and sequencing skills can cause.

- The child's attention should be fully gained when being given instructions. Also avoid giving too many instructions at one time as this can cause confusion.

- Specific activities that the child finds difficult may need some actual 'hands on' help: for example, organising paperwork and planning the flow of the day. See resources – IANSYST Ltd has valuable tools for children with organisational and sequencing issues.

- Multi-sensory reinforcement of instructions both verbally and visually – for example, print outs, information written up on board and the use of a keyboard – can be valuable. Ensure adequate information is taken down by the child to allow success in homework and other projects.

- Mind maps, extra planning time and a prepared format giving cues for what the child needs to consider when planning a project can assist.

- Ensure that the child has well-maintained writing and recording tools and strategies such as a 'see through' pencil case to allow quick checking of equipment. Also work topics should be colour coded and/or kept together in individual folders. The colour coding can be cross-referenced on a written timetable.

- The acquisition of keyboard skills prior to secondary school can provide an excellent strategy to enable a child with a recognised dyspraxia to organise their thoughts and ideas on paper as this enables efficient editing. Providing the child has gained competent keyboard skills of 20 to 25 words a minute, the use of a laptop can be gradually integrated into appropriate lessons with a view to using this strategy for higher level examinations.

- A watch with a clear face is vital: in secondary school a mobile phone or PDA (personal digital assistant) is valuable for reminders or main appointments. The child may need additional time for organising each transition in class.

● At home ensure that school clothes are laid out ready the night before and contents of the school bag checked against a visual timetable, the latter placed where the child can easily refer to it. Ensure updates are maintained for any changes.

Additional games and activities to facilitate organisation, sequencing and working memory

These can be integrated as part of a PE lesson or games.

● Obstacle races which can be adapted to provide as much variety as possible, involving left and right, through, round, up and over, to facilitate spatial organisation.

● Ball bouncing, catching, throwing games in pairs or groups taking turns – focusing on left and right, up and down, side to side and counting.

● Charades, mime and dance sequences.

● Hopscotch can be adapted for a variety of sequential activities, including hopping and jumping backwards, forwards and side to side.

● Card games such as Pairs, Pelmanism, Snap, Rummy, Knock Out Whist and Solitaire.

● Traditional games including Noughts and Crosses, Snakes and Ladders, dominoes, chess, strategic peg games, Kim's Game for working memory (see Happy Puzzle Company in the resources).

● Construction games and building games.

● Cartoon books/magazines for visual sequencing.

● Typewriting skills to a level of 20–25 words a minute for secondary school.

● Piano or other musical instruments.

● Horse riding, particularly involving indoor schooling.

● Activities under the direction of an occupational therapist for sensory motor integration.

Concentration and attention

What: definition and meaning

What?

- Focus, concentration and attention with the ability to sit quietly and still has been described as the result of a 'symphony' of integration in relation to a child's underlying sensory motor systems. Children with dyspraxia may lack integration as a result of an underlying developmental immaturity affecting their ability to concentrate and attend to the task in hand.

- The frontal area of the brain which supports cognition, impulse control, decision making, focus and attention may not have fully matured and integrated, making it particularly challenging for children whose schooling begins at a very early age.

- The maturity of the vestibular (balance) system is a key area in that when fully integrated it enables the child to be at the right level of 'arousal' and focus, with both sides of the brain working together for optimum learning.

- Sensory processing challenges may cause the child to lack concentration and attention due to difficulty in filtering out all the sensory information they receive through their tactile (touch), visual (looking) and auditory (listening) systems. These systems may be hypersensitive, affecting the child's ability to concentrate as a result of all the additional stimulation they are having to deal with.

So what: issues and challenges

So what?

- Children with dyspraxia or an underlying developmental co-ordination disorder can lack the cortical or brain inhibition for impulse and attention control and be easily taken off task. The child may be a 'dreamer' or easily distracted by their own thoughts.

- The child's underlying organisational and sequencing skills may be poor and their level of output and written work may be adversely affected.

- Children with sensory integrative dysfunction may also experience a reduced awareness of their own body position in space, affecting their level of concentration and focus.

◆ The child's touch system may be over- or underreactive, causing sensitivity to clothes textures and physical contact with other children, for example. This in turn can adversely affect their concentration on the task in hand in class.

◆ If the child has a heightened awareness of what is going on around them in terms of visual and sound distraction, especially in a busy classroom, the lack of concentration and attention can be exacerbated when the child is placed facing their peers as opposed to the focus of teaching.

◆ Vision and hearing may be heightened and acutely sensitive, causing distractibility (see Moro reflex in the next chapter). The child may be alert to sounds that are normally filtered out by others and not be able to distinguish the relevant incoming stimuli from the teacher or environment around them, causing them considerable distraction.

◆ It is important to ensure that the child has sufficient water throughout the day as dehydration can lead to lack of concentration. Ensure that the child has slow release high fibre foods, particularly at the beginning and middle of the day to maintain energy levels. Nutritional advice can also be sought, as some children who are low on essential nutrients such as omega 3s and iron, for example, can display poor concentration and attention.

◆ For those children with the more severe attention deficit (and hyperactivity) disorders – a condition sometimes seen overlapping with dyspraxia – medication is occasionally prescribed. The long-term effects of this are not yet clearly known, and support and advice on aspects of sensory processing can assist as an alternative technique.

Now what: practical strategies and ideas

- Whole class teaching is valuable where there can be shared quiet periods during the lesson to minimise distraction.

- The child's desk should face the teacher and the board to avoid turning between board and desk and the attendant distractions, particularly if the child's short-term auditory and/or visual retention is poor.

- Give time for planning and organisation of materials at the beginning of each task to avoid increasing the child's stress levels, as this can help them to settle and concentrate.

- Break down verbal and written instructions into simple steps, with a clear beginning, middle and end. Give reminders of what is to happen next. Minimise visual clutter on the desk and board where possible.

- Allow a multi-sensory approach to enable the child to use their best personal learning methods – for example, visual, auditory, tactile or kinaesthetic, or a combination for the younger child. If one channel for learning is weak, then others can be used in a compensatory manner to support learning skills.

- Minimise noise levels and movement around the child. Avoid placing a child with limited focus and attention span next to a window or in the main thoroughfare.

- Where possible, provide times of quiet where there can be complete attention on task in order to build up the ability to work for longer periods.

- Colour code different subject books, use a 'see through' pencil case so that materials can be seen at a glance and maintain the child's ability to feel in control.

- A child may be unable to transfer information across two planes: that is, between board (vertical) and paper (horizontal) – especially if eye movements are poor. It is helpful to put notes on the desk and/or allow extra time for recording information to limit stress and anxiety.

- Minimise pressure on the child and anxiety by giving positive feedback for the effort made during the lesson.

- Allow movement opportunities for children who are fidgety – for example, to give papers out – to ease any postural discomfort, which is common in children with an underlying co-ordination disorder.

- Allow a child with 'touch' sensitivity sufficient space to avoid unnecessary nudging and bumping as the child may overreact to physical contact.

- More unusually, if a child has occasional 'absences' and seems 'disconnected' from what is going on around them, resulting in a complete lack of response, this can sometimes indicate underlying mild seizure activity and should be monitored closely with a view to referring for a medical opinion. This is obviously different from being 'off task' or experiencing a general loss of attention or concentration.

Chapter 7

Primitive or baby reflexes

Overview

What: definition and meaning

What?

- Reflexes are early inbuilt automatic movement patterns, some of which start in the womb, and are a normal part of early development.

- These primitive automatic and involuntary movements help the developing baby to move through different stages of their physical development before birth, and play a particularly active part in the first two years or so of life.

- Reflexes are designed to have a protective role in the baby within the first few months of life after birth as well as facilitating the different stages of early motor development: for example, grasping, rolling, sitting, crawling and gradually progressing to standing.

- These primitive or baby reflexes are normally inhibited by the maturing brain within the first year or two of life, although they can be elicited in older children and adults, and may re-emerge in an older person as brain inhibition becomes weaker.

- If these early reflexes are not inhibited and integrated by the brain at the appropriate stage, they may have an adverse impact not only on a child's motor development and the refining of movement, but also on motor skill acquisition.

The following reflexes, if still present in the school-age child, may also have an adverse impact on their higher functioning skills and educational ability. One or more reflexes noted below may be seen in the child with a developmental co-ordination disorder or motor dyspraxia and may have a particular influence on a child's school attainment (Goddard, 1998; see also INPP under professional organisations):

- *Palmar reflex* – starts in womb and normally inhibited by 4 months.
- *Moro reflex* – starts in womb and normally inhibited by 3 months.
- *Asymmetrical tonic neck reflex (ATNR)* – starts in womb and normally inhibited by 6 months.
- *Symmetrical tonic neck reflex (STNR)* – starts at 6–9 months (pre-crawling) and normally inhibited by 9–11 months.

Palmar reflex

What: definition and meaning

What?

- The palmar reflex is a whole hand movement which emerges within the first 11 or 12 weeks after conception in the womb. Its function in part may be to help the baby maintain an automatic grasp – a 'safety' mechanism to enable the baby to hold onto the mother after birth.

- If the palm of a baby's hand is touched, stroked or has gentle pressure placed on it, the hand automatically closes into a fist with fingers bent. This response normally stays with the newborn baby during the first three months or so after birth.

- The palmar reflex should be automatically 'inhibited' within four to six months, allowing the baby to start to refine and isolate their finger and thumb movements in order to pick up and hold onto a small object with a 'pincer' grip using the opposing pads of the index finger and thumb.

- It takes a further few weeks for the baby to be able to release objects (hence the dropping of articles over the high chair) as this requires repetition and practice!

- Hand and mouth movements are strongly linked in the early years and are used for exploration of objects and the environment. In a newborn baby taking milk, a related 'kneading' movement of the hand may be noted as they suckle.

So what: issues and challenges

◆ Associated mouth or tongue movements may be observed when the child is writing, drawing or using scissors, particularly when the activity requires some resistance. This is due to the underlying retained hand and mouth neuro-developmental link. This associated movement is sometimes called 'overflow'.

◆ The child may have poor manual dexterity, as the whole hand grasp can limit independent finger and thumb movements. For example, in self-care activities, buttons, zips and scissor work will be harder for them and remain at a less mature stage of development.

◆ There may be lack of pincer grip, which can affect pen grip and control for cursive writing. The pen may be held in an immature position with the thumb lapped across the pen or with a general whole hand grasp making handwriting tiring and more effortful.

◆ Many children retain a palmar grasp if they are not assisted to refine their grip with fingers and thumb on the barrel of the pen, or move from a static pincer grip to a more dynamic active grip required for cursive writing. The immature pen grip does not, therefore, always reflect a developmental immaturity.

◆ The child may incur whole arm movements when writing, drawing or with general tool use, again making the activity far more effortful and extremely tiring when working for extended periods. They may be unwilling to write more than a sentence or two due to hand, arm, neck or back discomfort.

◆ The palms of the hand may be sensitive, making the child reluctant to engage in certain activities and withdraw from contact with certain materials and holding tools. Alternatively, some children with a palmar grasp often hold something in their hand at the expense of using that dominant hand to pick up an object.

◆ Speech and articulation may be poor and unclear due to the underlying link with hand and mouth that has not been automatically inhibited by the brain.

◆ Eating may be messy as the child does not have the musculature (oral motor control) for managing certain textures of food, and chewing takes longer.

◆ Certain foods may be harder to swallow; a stronger 'gag' reflex may be evident with a tendency for the child to choke. As a result, meals require more time and effort to deal with.

Now what: practical strategies and ideas

- Provide a board angled at 20 degrees, angled desk or folder, for a correct upper trunk and forearm position. This allows the wrist to extend and the hand to fall into a naturally flexed position with the fingers and thumb coming together in a pincer grip action on the barrel of the pen.
- Encourage the child to place their index, second finger and thumb onto the neck of the pen, using a thicker barrel with an integral textured grip if necessary – a grip normally achievable by year one (see resources).
- Exercises can be provided under the remit of a practitioner specialised in the field of reflex integration, or a therapist with understanding of reflex inhibition/integration. See the hand exercises below – incorporate grasp and release exercises, progressing to isolating finger and thumb movements.
- Advice can also be sought from an occupational therapist on activity ideas to help desensitise the child's hands.

Activities to promote pincer grip and isolation of finger and thumb movement

- Drawing on an upright chalkboard automatically assists the wrist and hand to fall into a pincer grip and correct wrist position (use chunky chalks).
- Encourage pincer finger and thumb grip using peg games, encourage wrist extension, and ensure that the child places the end pads of the index finger and thumb together when picking up a peg or a small object.
- Assist finger and thumb movements by incorporating pinch pots using clay and dough, activities using tweezers to pick up small objects, rolling marble/dice between finger and thumb, and turning pennies in the palm of the hand.
- Roll up a crepe bandage with one hand at a time using individual finger and thumb movements.
- Crumple up individual sheets of an old catalogue or telephone directory (use for target practice) – this provides strong 'grasp and release' exercise.
- Hit and keep a balloon in the air with a bat; once achieved, the child can then hit the balloon on alternate sides of the bat by turning the hand palm up and then back. Encourage the child to keep their elbow bent, to isolate forearm and hand movements.

- Playing the piano, flute or other musical instrument can help the child to refine and isolate individual finger and thumb movements.

- Keyboard training can be undertaken for children from the age of 9 or 10 if they experience ongoing difficulties with handwriting. A laptop can then be integrated into course work and examinations at secondary stage. Typewriting can be an additional remedial tool for finger and hand control, and in some children it can improve handwriting and spatial awareness in the recording of written and drawn information.

- Mouth control exercises – for example, blowing bubbles, suck and blow games – can be advised by a speech and language therapist, and additional advice can be sought from the same source if chewing, swallowing and speech articulation are adversely affected (see Royal College of Speech and Language Therapists under professional organisations).

Moro reflex ('flight, fight or fear' mechanism)

What: definition and meaning

What?

The Moro reflex is present as early as the first nine or ten weeks in the womb and is normally inhibited within two to four months in the young baby. It is elicited in response to an incoming, usually unexpected or unpleasant stimulus. It is there in part as a protective mechanism, and when stimulated can cause a whole body movement and stress reaction in the body. In response, the baby may startle, fling their arms out to the side, bend both legs up into a flexed position, take a large intake of breath prior to crying in a distressed manner.

The Moro reflex can be elicited by:

- A loud sound or noise – particularly if sudden and unexpected
- Bright light or other strong visual input or stimulation
- Sudden, unexpected movement or being poorly handled
- Pain or discomfort.

The consequences of a strongly retained Moro or 'flight, fight or fear' startle reflex may be observed in some children with autistic spectrum disorders who appear to be experiencing a high level of underlying stress. There may also be evidence of this reflex in some children with sensory processing difficulties who appear to be in a continual state of 'alert' with heightened sensory awareness.

So what: issues and challenges

♦ In the older child or adult it is commonly termed the 'flight or fight' response, and puts the individual on high 'alert' with their focus on incoming peripheral stimuli at the expense of concentration and attention. It may be present in children with attention deficit hyperactivity disorder. This state may be a result of raised cortisol in response to a heightened stress and anxiety level. This is a normal mechanism but not if the child remains in this state; it is hard for them to relax with their 'sympathetic' nervous system in chronic 'flight or fight' mode.

♦ The child may have very tense muscles, particularly around their shoulders and back, commonly termed 'armouring'. They may be extremely sensitive to touch, especially if approached unexpectedly from behind. They may be intolerant of certain materials and be hypersensitive to a range of incoming stimuli.

♦ The child may be very sensitive to light – particularly fluorescent lighting – and find white interactive boards or paper too bright, which can then affect their response in class. They may rub their eyes, and find reading and writing tiring (see also the vision and eye movement control section in Chapter 4 for other causes).

♦ Visual perceptual problems may be evident, and the child becomes what is called 'stimulus bound': they are unable to screen out or ignore irrelevant visual material within their field of vision and focus on the peripheral information at the expense of the task in hand.

♦ There may be some auditory (listening) confusion as the child may be sensitive to a range of incoming sounds and be unable differentiate relevant input such as the teacher speaking over and above the sound of their peers.

♦ The child may find sleep difficult due to their hypersensitivity to sound and the general bodily discomfort experienced. The slightest sound may bring them up out of sleep, resulting in sleep deprivation for them – and those around them. It is not uncommon for these children to have night terrors and fear of the dark due to a very creative imagination.

♦ There is often a dislike of change, transition and surprises, and the child may be rigid and controlling in their daily lives to avoid changes in routine and therefore what is, to them, additional stress.

♦ Balance and general co-ordination may be compromised, particularly in ball games. The child may turn their head or blink or avert their eyes when a ball is thrown to them as a result of the heightened protective mechanism and response.

◆ Motion sickness when travelling in a car is not uncommon. There may be fear of physical activity as a result of an underlying immature balance system.

◆ The child may have reduced stamina, energy and exercise tolerance, but at the same time may have periods of overactivity.

◆ The child may be emotionally volatile and overreact to situations and have a free-floating anxiety which does not have any obvious source but which is heightened when they are put under pressure.

◆ Intolerance to wheat, dairy and other foods may be present (see BANT and Nutrition Science under professional organisations) and the child's immune system may be weak, also resulting in allergies, skin sensitivity, ear and throat infections.

◆ The child's blood sugar may fluctuate more than other children's, causing them to become particularly irritable prior to meals.

◆ The child may react adversely to criticism as they lack an innate sense of integration; self-image may be poor and they may find it hard to adapt to new situations. Decision making can be difficult.

◆ The child may feel the need to control and manipulate situations in a desire to cope with their own anxieties and insecurities. Alternatively, they may demonstrate a high level of dependency on those around them due to the non-specific anxiety experienced.

Now what?

Now what: practical strategies and ideas

- A supportive structure and routine should be in place both at home and in school, with an understanding of the heightened stress levels the child may be experiencing.

- Plan a routine wherever possible; give the child verbal cues and a few minutes' warning for any transition or change of activity.

- Periods of quiet should be built into the school day and home routine (this assists most children). Whole class teaching is effective when group work is not underway, as it allows focus and attention due to extraneous sound being minimised.

- In class, minimise visual distractions where possible. Keep the environment immediately round the child uncluttered and organised.

- Lighting should be balanced and low level if the child's stress levels are to be lowered. Avoid fluorescent lighting and provide breaks from interactive whiteboards if the child's stress appears heightened.

- Coloured overlays or glasses with softer lenses may help to avoid the sharp contrast of black print on white paper or from interactive boards and computer screens. Give regular breaks when using technology.

- Provide positive feedback for effort made, avoid confrontation with a child who is stressed, and avoid shouting as this aggravates the situation.

- Build on the child's self-esteem as above, and ensure success in areas which may not be obvious initially. The child may be gifted in certain areas and find new confidence in a hobby or activity which fully absorbs them.

- A visual perceptual assessment may help to evaluate the child's interpretation of symbols and ascertain whether or not there are aspects of their focus that are out of balance.

- Provide some differentiation in PE and games for balance and co-ordination challenges. Be aware that the child may find excessive movement frightening, also heights and other challenging movement experiences such as walking along benches in PE, and using escalators and, to a lesser degree, lifts.

- Adapt ball games to build confidence, starting with throwing and catching balloons, larger foam balls and beanbags to avoid eliciting a 'startle' reaction.

- Be aware of the child's lack of stamina and exercise tolerance, or alternatively provide outlets for movement opportunities which can burn off excess energy.

- Allow the child to pursue activities which they find relaxing on their return home; provide them with a slow release high fibre snack prior to placing any further demands on them. Time out, in terms of relaxation, is important.

- Ensure that clothes are non-irritating and avoid scratchy labels to limit the amount of distracting extraneous demands on the child.

- Avoid 'learned helplessness' if the child has a high level of dependency; work towards success in small steps in activities, and allow extra time for the child to try activities hitherto avoided by them through fear of failure. They may be helped by taking responsibility in a task for someone less able. A child with this physiological make-up needs to feel valued and needs more reinforcement than others to prevent future inappropriate behaviours.

- Allow where possible a relaxing period before the child's bedtime; minimise any television programmes which can adversely affect the child's already charged up nervous system.

- Give time for the child to share their anxieties and plan positively for the next day. Plan positive and enjoyable activities for the child to look forward to at some part of the week.

- Advice should be sought from an occupational therapist experienced in sensory integration for a full evaluation of the child's 'sensory' profile and advice on a 'sensory diet' if issues continue to arise. A course of occupational therapy to address some of the above areas may be advisable.

- Children with allergies and intolerances may require the advice of a nutritional therapist to build up their immune system and to provide an adapted diet if necessary. Ensure that their blood sugar is maintained, avoiding sugary snacks and providing foods which have slow release nutrition. Also provide adequate drinking water throughout the day.

- A referral to an osteopath who can treat and reduce the child's sympathetic nervous system response may be valuable. This can assist the child's body to relax physiologically, and ensure there are no other bio-mechanical problems.

Further classroom strategies to minimise stress

The following are designed to help a child 'modulate' their behaviour and cope if they become overloaded with too much incoming stimuli.

■ Allow the child to stretch and take some deep breaths before settling down to work. Firm pressure, attained by sitting down, placing their weight onto straight arms with hands placed on the chair at either side of the body, can provide soothing feedback and help the child to modulate their behaviour.

■ Provide the child with an uncluttered desk in a less busy part of the classroom, but where they face the board and the focus of teaching.

■ At the start of a lesson, give the child sufficient opportunity to organise their equipment and writing materials to avoid any stress and tension. Any organisational difficulties can heighten stress and the fear of not being in control throughout the school day.

■ Provide clear instructions on the order of activities to assist the child to plan and stay on task appropriately. Gain eye contact where possible to help the child to focus.

■ Break down an activity into manageable steps for a child who has difficulty in processing and executing ideas on paper. Demonstrate an activity and provide visual and auditory cues where possible.

■ If the child is 'fidgety' and 'on the move', purchase a cushion which provides acceptable movement while sitting. Ensure that the chair height allows the child's feet to be placed firmly on the ground – weight bearing through the feet can provide firm pressure feedback. This in tandem with the adapted cushion can help the child to self-regulate their behaviour.

■ Where possible, alternate movement opportunities with periods of sitting and concentration – for example, by allowing the child to give out paper.

■ A visual timetable assists the child to have control over their day. Writing on a vertical chalkboard prior to writing on paper facilitates good posture, shoulder stability and increased feedback through the joints (proprioception).

■ The provision of an angled board (see Back in Action, Posturite and Philip and Tacey in resources) provides support and stability for the forearms and therefore improved hand and pen control.

- Water and high fibre snacks allowed at regular intervals can assist concentration. Chewing and eating (where appropriate) provides increased proprioception, which can help to calm the child. Nail biting may be a symptom of stress, but also a need for proprioceptive (calming) input – the two can be linked.

- Allow a strategy of time out if the child becomes overloaded with demands, frustrated or stressed – this can result in outbursts of anger.

- Be aware that some children find touch uncomfortable and distressing; allow personal space when moving around with other children to avoid a negative or inappropriate response.

Sleep strategies and ideas for the younger child

- Allow the child the opportunity for physical activity at the end of the school day to release any pent up energy or frustration. If the child has difficulty in settling down afterwards, ensure that they have calming time prior to preparing for bed.

- Avoid overstimulating activities such as tickling and chasing around unless on the child's terms, as this can easily overload a child with an immature nervous system, particularly if they have difficulty modulating their behaviour.

- Establish a manageable and practical bedtime routine – for example, a warm bath (lavender essence can be relaxing), a warm milk drink, and the opportunity to unwind, talk about the school day and any concerns they may have. Try, however, to end the conversation on an 'up' note!

- Children with dyspraxia often have a heightened perception of what is going on around them and may be very sensitive to visual information that would be 'filtered out' by another child. Ensure, therefore, that any unpleasant or unsettling viewing material is avoided on television and/or computer prior to bedtime.

- Ensure when reading a story that the content and illustrations are suitable and the storyteller's voice relaxed and low. The child can be helped to calm down by wrapping them around with a blanket or cuddling them, where appropriate, as firm pressure (not restraint) can soothe the nervous system (this takes about ten minutes).

- Soothing music can be played at bedtime. The 'Sound Health' series recordings have specially designed tapes to provide 'physiological' relaxation (see Learning Solutions in resources).

- Consider using blankets instead of a duvet, as these can provide soothing firm pressure feedback and some children prefer the weight of blankets and being tucked in. (This is a form of 'swaddling' for children – not restraint!) A sleeping bag is a good alternative for cosiness as long as the child can climb in and out easily. Where possible, place the bed against a wall to give a greater sense of security. Night clothing should ideally be made of cotton to provide extra comfort.

- A pillow placed in the bed along the child's back can provide firm, soothing pressure and reduce fidgeting. A hot water bottle with a soft cover can provide physical comfort.

- Check that the bedroom is not too light or too dark, too cold or too hot – keep the child's feet warm with bed socks if their temperature fluctuates.

- Additional blinds or lined curtains can be helpful during the summer if the child is sensitive to light, but with a small low-level nightlight to minimise fear of the dark if they have an overactive imagination.

- Glow-in-the-dark non-spill feeder cups can be purchased to put by the bed/cot for younger children.

- A simple prayer may help the child to feel safe and comforted.

Asymmetrical tonic neck reflex (ATNR)

What?

What: definition and meaning

An ATNR is an automatic whole body movement pattern which emerges in the womb and remains present up to approximately six months after a baby's birth. This reflex may play a part in the birthing process as it causes a whole body rotation movement pattern when the baby turns its head from one side to the other. It may, therefore, assist the body to rotate when the baby moves down the birth canal.

A 'fencing' or 'archery' posture can be observed in a small baby. It is elicited when the baby turns their head to one side – the arm and leg on that side stretch out and extend while the opposite arm and leg flex (bend). The opposite pattern occurs when the baby turns its head to face the other way. If this movement pattern is not automatically inhibited by the brain within the first year of life, the older child may have difficulty isolating head, body and arm movements in order to refine their arm and hand control. This particular reflex, if retained, appears to be linked with a lack of integration of both sides of the body (bilateral integration). Also it may limit the ability of the child to work across the midline of their body.

So what?

So what: issues and challenges

◆ The child may not have a clear hand dominance and may have a tendency to change hands during a task (mixed laterality). When undertaking more formal activities, the writing hand may not always be the most dextrous in some fine motor tasks (in other words, they are ambidextrous).

◆ Two-handed activities may be difficult for the child to co-ordinate – for example, in design and technology work, doing up laces and buttons, using a knife and fork – as they may not have a preferred leading or stabilising hand.

◆ The child may find it difficult to write and work across the body midline, and may twist or rotate their body or lean to one side to avoid it – this is usually done unconsciously, but more effort is incurred, making writing more onerous and less smooth.

◆ Excessive or fluctuating pressure on pen grips and paper may be noted: hand, arm and shoulder may ache due to the pressure exerted. (This may also be due to reduced body awareness and reduced feedback from the child's arms – see the section on proprioception in Chapter 3.)

◆ The child may have difficulty following a moving object in the horizontal plane with their eyes (visual tracking) and blink their eyes at their body midline due to poor integration of both sides of their body. Reading, including the ability to maintain line position and keep their place, may be affected. Words and letters may appear to 'jump around', or in some instances they may experience 'double vision'.

◆ There may be no clear eye dominance and the child is unsure which eye to use when looking through a telescope or camera.

◆ The child may have a fluctuating profile with regard to visual perception, particularly when matching symmetrical shapes and figures.

◆ Balance may be affected when the head is turned from side to side, as whole body rotation may be elicited by the head movement and throw the child off balance.

◆ Difficulty with reciprocal cross pattern movements may be experienced by the child during, for example, skipping, cycling and 'marching' patterns or when following a sequence of movements.

◆ When eating, the child may raise their elbows in the air at either side of the body as a result of the retained whole arm movement patterns. Use of knife and fork may be awkward with difficulty in cutting and controlling food.

Now what?

Now what: practical strategies and ideas

- Position the child facing the teacher and board or the focus of activity to limit the whole body rotation caused by turning their head. Handwriting and recording output will otherwise be adversely affected.

- Observe which hand the child tends to use as the leading hand for picking up and using a pen or object, and encourage the use of a consistent hand by placing activities to that side in the younger child.

- Encourage the child's wrist extension and dynamic tripod grip with the first two fingers and thumb placed on the barrel of the pen. A tripod grip allows use of the intrinsic, small muscles of the fingers and thumb for cursive writing. Exercises under the direction of an occupational therapist can assist the child to isolate head, trunk, arm, forearm, hand and finger movements to facilitate this skill.

- Provide the child with integral soft pen and pencil grips to ease pressure on the hand and fingers.

- Provide short breaks when writing for extended periods, 'shake' wrists and hands to relax and ease pressure, and provide an angled folder or angled posture board to rest the wrist on.

- Pen control is assisted by the child being placed symmetrically at the desk, with the height just below or at elbow level. Chairs which provide an upright position with lumbar support, allowing them to sit with their hips at 90 degrees for maximum stability, should be provided.

- Allow additional space on a shared table if the child tends to lean or shift to one side when writing to avoid crossing their body midline.

- Place the writing paper on the side of the child's writing hand; this can limit their need to write across the body midline.

- Provide the child with additional time to ease hand discomfort in tests and examinations.

- With the young child, practise tasks and activities which require both hands to be used together (symmetrical use); using both sides of the body together assists integration prior to working with cross pattern movements. Use cooking, collages, crafts, construction and lacing games.

- Use paper with carbon backing to check the pressure exerted on the paper, which the child can see and then adjust. Extra paper under the writing sheet can also ease the pen grip and hand pressure.

- Formal keyboard training may be required prior to or at secondary stage if handwriting continues to be a real issue. The introduction of a laptop may be recommended by an educational psychologist or occupational therapist into appropriate lessons for the child to ensure competency prior to any of the key examinations.

● It is important to check functional vision with an optometrist (see BABO under professional organisations) if the child is experiencing strain and difficulty with maintaining visual focus on the board, at the desk or for reading.

● A comprehensive visual perceptual and visual motor assessment may be required by an educational psychologist or occupational therapist (see professional organisations). Activities can also be provided by a suitably qualified occupational therapist, following a comprehensive assessment, with advice and strategies provided which can be shared with the school.

● Therapy programmes for reflex inhibition can be provided by appropriately qualified therapists to assist in facilitating higher level functional skills (see INPP under professional organisations).

Symmetrical tonic neck reflex (STNR)

What: definition and meaning

- A retained STNR may be present in children with a developmental co-ordination disorder or motor dyspraxia.

- It is one of a cluster of reflexes or involuntary automatic movement patterns, some of which emerge in the womb. The STNR normally presents after birth around the first six months of a baby's life.

- This reflex, which is part of normal physical movement development, helps the child to move into a four-point kneeling position prior to establishing crawling.

- If the reflex is retained after nine or ten months of life – around the usual period for crawling – it may have an adverse or 'blocking' effect on the progression of the child's motor development, affecting, for example, their ability to move forward and integrate left and right sides of the body for crawling.

- Crawling (using arms and legs in a reciprocal movement pattern) is an activity which may assist in maturing and integrating the following aspects of development and sensory motor integration:

  (a) The body's ability to perform reciprocal movement patterns and integration of both sides of the body (bilateral integration).

  (b) Eye and hand co-ordination and adjustment of eye movements near and far.

  (c) Postural stability – shoulder and hip strengthening while weight-bearing through shoulders and hips.

  (d) Feedback back through firm pressure for body position awareness (proprioception).

  (e) Wrist, finger and thumb extension (web space) for manipulation.

So
what?

So what: issues and challenges

◆ The child may have never crawled using both sides of the body in a reciprocal movement pattern on all fours, preferring to bottom shuffle or 'commando' crawl.

◆ Where the STNR is retained, it can be activated when the child bends their head over their work at school, and their arms may automatically flex as a result of the linked movement which has not fully dissociated. At the same time the child's legs may have a tendency to straighten. The opposite pattern of movement can also occur, and the child may find whole body extension or flexion difficult, especially when sitting for long periods in a flexed position.

◆ As a result, it may be difficult for the child to maintain an upright sitting posture at a desk or table. They may 'prop' their head on their hand at the expense of stabilising their work or using both hands together, fidget, wrap feet behind chair legs, prefer to sit on their feet, and need change their position frequently. When in class the child may sit with their arms crossed and their legs stretched out in front of them (this posture can look oppositional). They may even try to stand up to write or lean back and write with their arms extended in an attempt to ease their postural discomfort.

◆ The child may find sitting cross-legged on the floor difficult and prefer to sit in a 'W' position with their knees bent under them, feet out to the side.

◆ They may dislike and avoid writing as it requires extra effort. Poor letter formation and excessive pressure on the paper may be observed, and they may break pencil points frequently. Discomfort in the neck, back and writing hand may be experienced.

◆ Homework can become a battlefield with the child. It may be rushed and the child may find it difficult to complete.

◆ The child may lose their place when copying work from a board or book in part due to difficulty with eye movement control and adjustment from one place to another (see advice on optometrist below).

◆ Reading difficulties may be experienced.

◆ Difficulty with maintaining attention may be experienced, with trouble focusing on a task. They may daydream, lose attention quickly, be easily distracted and fiddle with everything on their desk.

◆ Co-ordination challenges may be experienced by the child, especially between the upper and lower parts of the body, and they may have trouble with cycling, skipping, marching, running, catching and throwing; they may avoid certain sports as a result. Symmetrical activities such as skiing may not be a problem, and the child may be competent overall in these areas.

◆ When swimming using the breast stroke, the child may find it difficult to keep their head above water when bending their arms due to the linked head and arm flexion patterns.

Now what: practical strategies and ideas

Now what?

- Allow some stretching and movement prior to sitting for extended periods, but also short appropriate movement breaks during the writing session to ease mechanical discomfort.

- The child may require a physiotherapy or osteopathic check to ensure that their spine is in alignment if they complain of back and neck discomfort when writing for extended periods.

- Encourage the use of an angled board or folder when writing to ensure that the upper body is as upright as possible – when the head is bent over the desk, the weight on the neck can change from approximately 4 kilos to 14 kilos due to the pull of gravity.

- Be aware that handwriting and schoolwork may be more laborious for these children than for their peers. Ensure that the child is facing the focus of teaching and notes are provided on the child's handwriting side where possible.

- Provide the child with integral pen grips to ease pressure as well as short breaks with additional time for written work as appropriate.

- Ensure a good visual line for copying from the board. Give the child time to adjust their vision from board to book.

- Check functional vision/eye movements with an optometrist to ensure eye strain and visual tracking are not a problem. This needs to be in addition to an optician's report (see BABO under professional organisations). Eye exercises moving eyes from near to far points and back may be helpful.

- Good postural support needs to be provided for homework, with opportunities for five-minute movement breaks from the work station. A higher stool and raised work surface or an angled cushion (Move 'n' Sit – see Back in Action in resources) may ease mechanical discomfort.

- Provide enhanced access to computers and/or a laptop for extended written assignments.

- Assess for the use of a personal laptop if the issues are causing real concern with regard to a mismatch between writing output and the child's innate skills. For example, keyboard programme information is available from IANSYST Ltd (see resources), and access should be sought for formal keyboard training to be integrated into school lessons prior to secondary school examinations.

- Upper and lower body co-ordination may be difficult, so some allowance should be given for games and PE activities which incorporate reciprocal movement patterns.

- Exercises to encourage total flexion/extension patterns may be helpful. A remedial exercise programme may be advised by an occupational therapist. For example, extending the full body in a slow stretch and then full flexion of the body, rolling it up into a ball and then stretching out, moving from the crouch position into a 'star' position. Exercises should be undertaken for ten to fifteen minutes, two or three times a week, and where possible be built into PE sessions.

- Specific swimming training may be required to assist the child to overcome the retained whole movement patterns of upper and lower body incurred by the retention of this reflex.

Activity ideas to assist large motor and reflex integration

All motor activities should be undertaken SLOWLY AND UNDER CAREFUL SUPERVISION.

- Wall push-ups. Stand at arm's length from the wall, heels down on the ground. With straight arms and wrists extended, place palms of hands flat against the wall while keeping back straight. Take weight onto hands, bend arms slowly and straighten – feel stretch on back of legs as arms are bent. Repeat five to ten times.

- Stand with arms out to sides; slowly turn body a full circle and then turn the other way. Repeat two or three times but monitor for dizziness and/or unsteadiness.

- Lie on stomach and lift head, chest, arms and legs off the ground as straight as possible for up to 30 seconds (if over the age of 7).

- Lie on back, reach out for and touch foot with hand on same side of the body. Change sides and repeat five times. Touch foot with opposite hand five times, change to other hand and foot and repeat five times.

- Lie on back, lift opposite legs and arms one at a time and then together, change sides and repeat. Lift alternate arms and legs in sequence. As one arm or leg is raised, lower the other one.

- Lie on back and reach for beanbag or half-kilo weight on opposite side of the body, pick up and place it on near side. Repeat with the other arm five times.

- Lie on back with arms and legs straight. Turn head to the left while slowly bending left arm and leg, then relax. Turn head to the right – slowly bend right arm and leg, then relax. Repeat both five times.

- Kneel on all fours, place left hand on left hip, turn the head to the left and lift and straighten right leg in the air, hold position to count of five. Repeat on opposite side. This may take considerable effort at first. *Work within the child's comfort zone in this and all the other advisory activities.*

- Lie in an extended position, roll slowly one way and then back again across floor mats.

- Kneel on all fours; with helper pushing against shoulders, crawl as far as possible and back again.

■ Sitting cross-legged, plan a sequence of movements to include 'cross pattern' clapping movement patterns incorporating working across the body midline. The child can make up or follow different sequences.

■ Lie on top of a 'peanut' shaped therapy ball and gently rock onto extended arms and hands; allow arms to bend slowly, straighten and then roll back again. Stretch legs out straight when rolling over onto hands.

■ Sit back to back against a large therapy ball with a partner – gently bounce back against the ball to gain firm pressure feedback while maintaining the sitting position.

■ Sit with knees bent and pass a foam ball in figure of eight around and under legs, ensuring that the ball is passed across from one side to the other in order to work across the body midline. Take turns to plan different short sequences.

■ Sit in a circle. Make a shape with hands and fingers, and 'pass it on' to the next person – each child to think up a pattern.

■ Make a shape with the body and 'pass it on' to the next person – involve every child in the motor planning of the shape by giving each of them a chance to think up and demonstrate a new position.

■ Dough, lacing and peg games can enhance pincer grip and isolate finger and thumb movement.

Chapter 8

Daily living (self-care) skills

Independence in toileting

What: requirements for managing the toileting process

What?

- Awareness of body and limb position in space (proprioception).
- Reasonable range of arm movements.
- Manual dexterity and grip, the ability to manipulate fastenings.
- Tactile (touch) awareness when hands are outside the field of vision.
- Reasonable postural stability and balance.
- Basic upper arm strength for pulling trousers or underwear up and down, ability to hold dress or shirt up, and balance on toilet.
- Ability to reach toilet roll easily, manipulate paper, balance, ensure clothes are out of way.

So what: issues and challenges

So what?

- ◆ The child may have a reduced sense of their own body scheme and limb position in space, adversely affecting their ability to carry out the activity effectively.
- ◆ The child may not be able to sense where their arms and hands are when outside their visual field (reduced proprioception).
- ◆ The presence of retained immature reflex movement patterns may affect manual dexterity and the child's ability to handle and manipulate toilet paper effectively.
- ◆ Balance may be poor when turning round or leaning over. The child may experience a feeling of being unsafe if their feet are not supported on the ground or on a small footstool due to postural instability.

Now what?

Now what: practical strategies and ideas

- Inform the school's special needs co-ordinator of possible problems to enable appropriate monitoring.
- Assist the child to follow the same routine where possible at home, which can also be translated into the school situation.
- Allow enough time for toilet routine – pressure will only aggravate the problem and create anxiety in the child.
- With a younger child, practise the routine at home, gradually reducing help as independence improves.
- Make sure the younger child's feet are supported when sitting at the toilet to provide postural security. If necessary provide a stable foot rest.
- Use a toilet seat insert for the younger child if postural stability or balance is poor.
- Toilet paper must be close enough with the use of a holder which allows sections of paper to be pulled off one or two handed.
- Disposable cleansing tissues can assist and be used in conjunction with toilet roll and kept by the child for use at school.
- Routinely reinforce the need for the child to wash and dry their hands properly.
- Where a child is reluctant, provide a star chart at home to note progress and effort made. Reward at the end of the week for successful outcome as this can be motivating.
- Give praise and positive reinforcement for effort made, even if end results are not perfect (yet)!

Dressing skills

The following are approximate age guidelines for dressing skills.

At 1 year:
- Child can start to join in and co-operate when being dressed by holding out a foot or arm to push into shoe or armhole.
- Can pull loose socks off and start to pull at shoes to take them off.
- Can take or pull hat off.
- Some awareness of nappy soiling from approximately 15 months and may indicate this to the carer.

At 2 to 3 years:
- Can remove a simple item and shoes if article is undone or loose.
- Can place their foot into trousers, but not usually aware of correct leg.
- May help to push clothing down at the toilet.
- Can find armholes in a simple top with slight prompts and supervision.
- Will try to put on socks, also shoes and boots, providing balance is reasonable.
- Can put on a simple jumper or coat with help.

At 3 to 4 years:
- Starts to put on top – sometimes the wrong way round or inside out – may need help to position it and then take it off.
- Can pull lower looser garments down for toilet and, when changing, take them off.
- Should manage large buttons and can put shoes on with adapted fasteners, but not always on the right foot.
- Zips can be pulled up but needs help to insert the shank first.
- Starts to put clothes on the right way round with some exceptions.
- Fastenings become easier, including buttons and undoing front fastening zips.
- Gloves with fingers need help but can manage fingerless gloves and own boots.
- Can now dress but with prompting and supervision.

At 4 to 5 years:

■ Should be able to achieve most fastenings with some help and guidance, including a zip.

■ Can put socks on correctly and shoes with easy fastening should be manageable with a little supervision.

■ Now technically old enough to manage laces!

■ Should know the spatial orientation, back and front, of a garment.

■ The child is on the way to independent dressing with prompts and some practical help.

At 5 to 6 years:

■ Now should be able to put garments on the right way round and dress themselves unsupervised.

■ Also able to tie knots, including behind their back outside their visual field.

What: requirements for competent dressing skills

■ A reasonable sense of one's own body scheme and position of body parts (proprioception).

■ A spatial awareness of personal body scheme in relation to the surrounding environment and clothes – what is up and down, side to side, in front and behind.

■ Adequate sense of touch (tactile) feedback – not over- or undersensitive.

■ Reasonable hand and eye co-ordination, especially for fine motor tasks.

■ Good balance and postural stability to be able to stand on one leg when putting pants or socks on and taking them off.

■ Ability to work across the body midline when reaching across to position clothes and tuck them in.

So what: issues and challenges

◆ The child may have a poor sense of their body scheme and be unsure which way to put their clothes on and how. They cannot organise their clothes when outside their visual field, leave clothes untucked, and generally untidy and out of place.

◆ Clothes may be put on back to front or inside out by the child; extra time may be needed to get clothes on properly. Sequencing, planning and general organisation for getting dressed in the morning, or for gym and sports, are difficult and frustrating for both child and supervisor. The child may seem 'all fingers and thumbs'.

◆ The child may be touch sensitive and, as a result, materials, labels, fastenings, waistbands may feel prickly and uncomfortable. The child will be constantly adjusting their clothes or fidgeting very often at the expense of focus on a main task.

◆ Alternatively, the child may lack touch sensitivity and be unaware of clothes hanging off their shoulders, poorly tucked in or not positioned correctly. They may not notice if shoes/boots rub blisters.

◆ The child may become frustrated with fastenings and zips and become angry at themselves and those around them when struggling with getting dressed. They may avoid getting dressed and try to divert from the job in hand.

◆ Standing to get dressed may be difficult for the child if their static and moving balance is weak, their muscle tone 'low'.

◆ The child may not be able to co-ordinate both sides of the body properly for use, and have difficulty reaching across the middle of their body to put on and adjust clothing.

Now
what?

Now what: practical strategies and ideas

- It may assist the younger child with dyspraxia to engage in 'push pull' games and activities or 'bounce' on a therapy ball prior to getting dressed, as this will give them increased sensory feedback and enhance their body position awareness (proprioception).

- At home, assist the child to prepare and lay out their clothes the night before. Establish a routine with drawers labelled correctly for socks, shirts and underclothes. Place clothes correctly in position, face down on the bed, to help the sequence and orientation of the garments in relation to the child's body.

- Provide a chair which offers more stability than a soft bed to limit balance difficulties; the clothes can then be placed on the bed in front of the child in a daily routine.

- Provide clothes with minimal resistance to being pulled on, such as trousers with elasticated waists. Put loops inside waistbands to pull up on if hand grip is weak; sew in elastic shanks for sleeve buttons which can remain done up but expand to allow the child to push their hands through. A circular clip such as a key-ring can be inserted into a zip to improve the child's grasp.

- Use large textured buttons for easier manipulation where possible. Use 'tube' or heelless socks – fold or roll down sock and insert toe. Talcum powder can help socks to slip on and off if feet get hot and sticky. Purchase shoes with adapted but normal looking fastenings.

- Provide natural materials where possible, remove scratchy labels, and avoid tight waistbands to limit any overt touch sensitivity. Avoid harsh detergents, use a natural clothes softener.

- Prompt the child to check in a mirror before leaving the room to ensure clothes are in position.

- Provide a hook on the door to hang large garments on, ready for the morning. Ensure outdoor clothes are placed on a hook in the correct position at the front door the night before to avoid further frustration, with a set place for shoes and boots.

- Allow the child additional time to get dressed and undressed at school for games and PE by letting them go first in the queue.

- Advice and practical help for daily living and self-care skills can be sought from an occupational therapist if the child continues to struggle with dressing. The therapist can also advise on core stability and balance exercises.

Chapter 9

Additional exercises, activities and therapy

Activities to strengthen trunk, shoulders and hips, and to increase body awareness

For a child who lacks confidence in the use of equipment, use the playground or gym when it is quieter with fewer children to compete with. Give positive encouragement and praise for any effort the child makes. Ensure success with the 'just right' level of activity, which may mean that they need to start with a simple movement activity, building up to an age-appropriate skill level over a few sessions.

- Child lies on stomach over large 'peanut' therapy ball and takes their weight on their extended hands through slightly bent elbows and wrists – then slowly straightens arms, lifts head, and extends body and legs. Child gently rolls forward onto fully bent elbows, lowers head and shoulders towards ground, then extends up again. Child repeats several times if comfortable with this.

- Note: do not attempt 'wheelbarrow' activities with weight of child's body supported through arms and legs, particularly if child's joints are hyper mobile or if muscle tone and general postural stability are weak. Child should always have support under their body.

- Provide 'peanut' ball for child to sit on with legs either side and gently bounce. Once feeling balanced, child can throw and catch beanbag or balloon while balancing on ball.

- Child sits back to back with partner, pushing against them – they lean forwards and backwards in a smooth and symmetrical manner, taking turns to take weight of other person's back.

- Try same activity but with large therapy ball placed between backs of partners. They should maintain upright position and a balance of force between them.

- Child kneels in upright position and maintains position while throwing and catching large foam ball or patting balloon backwards and forwards with partner. Depending on level of ability, they may progress to throwing and catching a beanbag.

■ Child kneels opposite partner and pushes against their extended hands while holding body in upright position; they must try to maintain stability.

■ Wall 'push ups' – child stands at arm's length from wall. With straight arms and extended wrists, they place palms on wall, keeping body and legs straight, and bend elbows and slowly lean towards wall, then extend arms slowly until pushed back into upright position. Child starts with four or five pushes and builds up number as shoulders and back become stronger. When done correctly, there should be a gentle pull on the calves.

■ For younger children, make up obstacle course which encourages crawling (reciprocal movement patterns), changes of direction, stretching, balance and body awareness feedback.

■ Provide play dough for child to knead and work. Ensure there is plenty of resisted two-handed activity to build up shoulder strength – this can be achieved by child standing at a table and pushing down on dough.

■ These activities are advisory only and the safety of the children is the responsibility of the supervising carer. Activities should always be undertaken under strict supervision with provision of suitable matting to provide a soft landing!

'Christmas Activity Box': therapy ideas for primary school children

These activities provide intervention for the following areas and can be adapted according to each child's level of ability:

- Postural stability and strength
- Muscle strength for both gross and fine motor skills
- Static and moving balance
- Ball and targeting skills
- Bilateral integration – working both sides of the body together and in alternating patterns of movement
- Working across the body midline
- Body scheme and position awareness
- Motor planning and organisation of movement
- Eye and hand co-ordination
- Manual dexterity and fine motor skills
- Motor and visual spatial skills
- Sequencing and left and right orientation
- A multi-sensory approach using body movement, touch, vision, hearing and speech
- Fun and the 'just right' challenge: positive praise should be given for effort as opposed to the end result.

Materials required:
- Children's safety scissors
- Paper, glue
- Adhesive tape for marking out lines on a level floor
- Beanbag (can be made up with dried beans sewn into different shapes such as a triangle, square and circle – can be numbered or lettered)
- Baton
- Hoop
- Balloons – ideally large size but blown up to three-quarter size for strength

- A foam ball and tennis ball
- Range of coloured straws – large width for cutting and threading
- Self-adhesive stickers
- Coloured pencils and thick marker for lines for scissor work
- Tracing paper
- Carbon paper
- Graph paper
- Lace with a hard tip
- Dough – made to recipe
- Dice.

The activities will require:
- Allocated space, up to three times a week
- Floor that allows lines to be taped on it
- Wall to bounce a ball against
- 'Record' book to note strengths and difficulties and any changes.

The materials should be provided in a kit and set aside from general toys and activities. The equipment should be used constructively for a 10- to 15-minute session at least three times a week. Ideally each session should incorporate all of the following:

- A fine motor manual task
- Balance, hopping or jumping practised two or three times
- Activities to work opposite sides of the body together.

Activities for balance, postural stability and bilateral integration

The child can be assisted to balance by holding hands with assistant, progressing to independent balance over the run of exercises.

Tape a 4-metre line on the ground. The child to:
- Walk placing feet alternately in front of each other along the line – slowly and carefully. It may assist the child if they are told to fix their vision on a point on the opposite wall.

- Slowly walk along the line, heel and toes placed touching each other along the line. Assistant to help the child if necessary.
- Move down the line, placing one foot at a time on opposite sides of the line – child to hold assistant's hand if needed.
- Place two feet together, jump both feet apart on either side of the line and then back together again, alternating the action to the end of the line.

Tape a 1-metre by 1-metre right-angled cross on the ground

- With feet together jump in a clockwise direction in and out of the four different sections until back to the start. Repeat two or three times at a steady pace.
- Jump from side to side in the different planes – left to right, right to left, up and down, down and up. The assistant reinforces the exercise verbally to support spatial awareness.
- Jump backwards over the lines landing with feet together round all four sections.
- Hop using preferred leg – in a *clockwise* direction into all four sections.
- Hop using opposite leg – in an *anti-clockwise* direction into all four sections.

Activities for ball and targeting skills, eye and hand co-ordination

These activities use a beanbag, foam ball and tennis ball. Always allow the child a few initial practices. The child to:

- Kneel facing a partner, sitting back onto feet, throw or roll foam ball to each other using both hands – up to 10 to 15 times slowly and methodically, watching the ball as it rolls. The distance between the partners can be adjusted according to their skill level.
- Repeat activity, but one-handed for throwing or rolling, using the dominant (handwriting) hand.
- Stand to throw and catch foam ball two-handed.
- Repeat actions using a beanbag until successful (may need to start at a metre distance and gradually increase space).

- Practise bouncing a tennis ball with dominant hand until it can be caught successfully with both hands at least six times in a row.
- Stand between 1 and 2 metres from a wall, throw the ball and allow it to bounce and be caught using two hands together, up to 10 or 15 times.

Baton activities for postural stability and trunk strengthening, bilateral integration and peer interaction

- Sitting cross-legged opposite a partner and with two hands placed on a baton, pull backwards and forwards in a rhythmic manner, as though rowing a boat, taking the partner's weight as they lean back. Ensure that some resistance is felt through the arms and shoulders.
- Kneel opposite partner, sit on heels and gently push and pull on the baton while maintaining an upright position.
- Kneel up on one knee, push and pull gently against the baton, change legs and repeat.

Hoop activities for bilateral integration using reciprocal movement patterns, working across the body midline, sequencing, counting and peer interaction

- Standing opposite partner, hold a hoop horizontally, placing both hands palms down on the hoop. Move hoop through hands to the left by placing the right hand across and over the other hand, releasing it and then grasping it again – 10 or 15 times slowly. Repeat activity, this time moving the hoop through the hands to the right.
- Standing opposite partner, turn hoop slowly in a vertical position by placing one hand above the other on the hoop while moving it through the hands. One partner will be moving the hoop up and over, and the other will move it downwards. Then reverse the pattern of movement by feeding the hoop in the opposite direction. Ensure that fingers are extended when letting go of the hoop.

Balloon for eye and hand co-ordination, timing, force, sequencing and counting

- Keep the balloon up in the air for as long as possible with both hands, individually or with a partner.
- Keep the balloon up in the air for as long as possible using a baton or table tennis bat with the dominant hand, then with both hands together.
- The balloon can be filled with a handful of lentils to give sound feedback and make it a little heavier.

Dice for fine motor skills, manipulation, isolating finger movements, assisting pen control and manual dexterity

- Manipulate a dice between finger and thumb, moving it up to the tip of each finger and back to the palm. Practise with each finger one at a time.
- Place a dice in the palm of the writing hand, call out any number up to six, then manipulate the dice using fingers and thumb to the correct number.
- Throw the dice, noting the number on the dice, then hold up the same number of fingers (up to five, including the thumb!) shown on the dice; try to keep the remaining fingers bent in the palm of the hand.

Straws/scissors for early scissor skills, fine motor manipulation and oral motor activities

Note: safety scissors should be used, under supervision.

- Cut several straws into pieces. Keep elbows at sides and thumb on top when manipulating scissors.
- Thread cut pieces of straw onto shoelaces or fine cord.
- Use straw pieces to make a picture with glue.
- Card cutting following different width lines, shapes, angles and patterns that have been pre-drawn or printed. Start with thicker, straight lines, and progress to curved and angled finer lines. Ensure the thumb is placed in the top hole of the scissors.
- Using a simple animal or pattern shape cut from newspaper, blow the shape through a straw along the floor and over a taped line to denote

the finish. Blowing games can help with extension of the body while sucking games help with body flexion.

■ Bubble blowing can also be used for promoting oral motor muscle strength and control of breathing in tandem with other activities under the direction of a speech and language therapist.

Self-adhesive stickers, tracing, carbon and graph paper for fine motor and manipulation skills, spatial orientation on paper

■ Use stickers to make own picture designs. Assistant provides the child with support to encourage imagination and also success with manipulation.

■ When tracing, choose favourite pictures and outlines to trace and then colour in. This activity can provide successful results for children who find free drawing difficult.

■ Place carbon paper between two sheets of paper; write or draw on the top sheet to practise creating an even pressure on the bottom sheet.

■ Graph paper is useful for writing the body of a letter or number, playing 'hangman', colouring in squares to make different patterns, copying a prepared design – progress from simple to more complex shapes.

Dough recipes for strengthening muscles of the hand and improving manual dexterity

Encourage the child to participate in this activity for five or ten minutes each session.

■ Make up dough as part of the activity – alternatively, readymade pastry can be used and then made or cut into shapes to be baked.

■ Squeeze and roll out dough using both hands, make up coil or slab pots from cut-out rectangular or square shapes.

■ Create own designs in dough and make animal models, coil or slab pots.

■ Roll out dough and mark patterns on it using everyday implements such as either end of a fork or spoon, then dry and paint.

Specific activities can be advised by an occupational therapist.

Horse riding ideas for the child with dyspraxia and allied conditions

- Horse riding provides firm pressure feedback (proprioception) through the sensory systems, and when undertaken in a calm and steady way can assist a child to relax. Body scheme and limb position awareness is alerted, assisting sensory integration.

- If the child is sensitive to movement (overresponsive), all activity on the pony should be monitored and taken at a much slower pace initially, in order for them to feel safe – make the experience dignifying, the 'just right' challenge and fun.

- Faster trotting in a large circle is stimulating for the child; this and also turning in different directions will stimulate their balance systems and help a sense of integration with the firm pressure feedback from the pony, providing the child feels safe and supported.

- If the child is movement seeking with an underresponsive system, they will be able to tolerate much more movement and activity in horse riding, but again they need to be closely monitored.

- Changing direction at a walking pace, and more particularly when trotting, helps to stimulate the child's balance systems and in turn to mature a rider's postural reactions and ability to adjust their body in space.

Horse riding can assist the following areas to develop:
- Postural reactions and adjustments and body stability.
- Head control.
- Muscle strengthening of the trunk and upper body, arms and legs.
- Release of tight muscles, particularly in the lower limbs, with the assistance of gravity.
- A sense of one's body position in space and general increased sense of 'self'.
- Relaxation through firm pressure feedback.
- General co-ordination of muscles including eye and hand co-ordination.
- Strengthening and helping to sustain grip.
- Functional eye movement control.
- Integration of both sides of the body and helping the child to work across the midline of their body.
- Sequencing, letter and number work when used in the riding lesson.

- Visual and motor spatial awareness, a general sense of orientation in space – may help to overcome dyslexic tendencies with regard to balance input, sequencing and spatial orientation, for example.
- General planning and organisation of movement.
- Communication and vocalisation.
- Feeling in control of a situation when supported appropriately.

Horse riding can provide sensory integration input for the following areas:

- Touch
- Smell
- Hearing
- Body position awareness
- Balance systems
- Vision.

Horse riding can also provide positive input for:

- Cognitive skills
- Emotional connection
- Self-confidence
- Concentration and focus
- Self-discipline
- Care and compassion for animals
- FUN.

Practical tips prior to a lesson

- Ideally ask the riders and their carers to stand a little way from the mounting block and then instruct each rider to come up one at a time with their carer. This enables the rider getting on the pony to know who is actually giving the instructions and support to them and avoids confusion caused by background noise.
- One person at a time should give verbal guidance to avoid auditory confusion in the rider. The child otherwise may not know who is giving the instructions or whom to listen to.
- Use a low and well-modulated but clear voice to soothe any initial anxieties in the child, particularly in the initial stages.

- Being assisted and moved up into the saddle may be alarming for some riders with immature balance systems, and may result in some stress responses such as hand flapping and loud vocalising.

- Give the rider time to settle and relax down into the saddle. If safe, allow the child's legs to rest down either side of the pony for a few seconds before assisting the feet into the stirrups.

- Assist the rider to place their hands down onto the pony and feel a sense of their connection with it, before asking them to follow instructions.

- Describe the pony – for example, its name and colour – so the rider is able to focus on the animal as opposed to any fears they may be experiencing.

- Lead the pony away from the mounting block and prepare the rider with some simple exercises while the rest of the group are still mounting their ponies.

Exercises on the pony prior to the group activity

A selection of the activities below can be made depending on the rider and the time available.

- Remember that ideally only one person at a time should be giving instructions to avoid confusion for the rider.

- After ensuring that the horse or pony is clear of any other animal, the rider can then undertake some simple exercises.

- Gently take the hands of the rider and explain what is going to happen, then assist them to give their arms a gentle shake to ease any tightness and tension in the shoulders. The rider should then relax their arms back onto the pony's neck or saddle.

- Encourage the rider with clear spoken prompts to give their arms a good stretch – ideally up above the head – gently two or three times. Then ask and assist the rider to stretch their arms out to the sides and back again, two or three times.

- The rider rests their hands onto the reins and then leans forward and reaches towards the horse's ears with both hands (providing the horse tolerates this well), then rests back into the saddle.

- Encourage the rider to cross their arms across their body and give themselves a 'big hug' – then stretch their arms out in front of them and repeat the big hug, reaching across their body midline.

- Assist or ask the rider to cross their arms out in front of them and place either hand on the opposite side of the pony's neck – cross and uncross the arms two or three times (integration of both sides of the body).

- The rider places their hands on the front of the saddle – encourage them to look up to the roof, gently stretching and extending their necks, then to turn their heads to look at one side helper and then the other side helper. (This helps to isolate head and body movements and to provide neck, back and shoulder release. In addition, it provides social interaction and preparation for the ride.)

- Rider pats the pony and then prepares to join the shared lesson.

For more information see the Riding for the Disabled Association's website (RDA under professional organisations).

Afterword

This book has gradually expanded in size from its original conception, but with a condition like dyspraxia there are endless permutations relating to this fascinating subject. Nevertheless, it is hoped and believed that this book will enhance the understanding of dyspraxia, and as a result improve many children's lifestyles and provide some extra 'stepping stones' for a successful future.

It is commonly observed in the Christmas Children's Clinic that many adults in the so-called 'normal' population have unrecognised dyspraxic profiles, struggling through life but not understanding why it is harder work for them than for others around them. They normally cope by providing their own strategies (sometimes by avoidance of a task), ensuring that this hidden and little understood condition does not limit their everyday functioning – but always at a cost. This is the crux of the matter: something needs to be done for the children whose sensory motor challenges are adversely impacting on their everyday lives. This is when a comprehensive assessment along with customised profile and strategies can be invaluable. It is hoped that this book has unlocked some of the answers to the questions that many parents, teachers and children ask: What? So what? Now what?

Jill Christmas, 2009

Resources

Note: all websites included here are correct at January 2009, but may be subject to change.

Ann Arbor Publishers Ltd – www.annarbor.co.uk – assessment materials and resources for special educational needs.

Anything Left Handed – www.anythingleft-handed.co.uk – help for left-handed children information page.

Back in Action – www.backinaction.co.uk – posture pack – a portable writing slope, seat wedge with pencil/paper storage and carry handle, Move 'n' Sit cushions.

Better Books – www.betterbooks.com – a range of excellent publications relating to developmental conditions.

British Dyslexia Association – www.bdadyslexia.org.uk – help with handwriting information page.

Come Unity – www.comeunity.com – articles to help your child with sensory integration issues.

Happy Puzzle Company Ltd – www.happypuzzle.co.uk – fun and educational activities and resources for schools.

IANSYST Ltd – www.dyslexic.com – whole range of IT and allied resources for children with dyslexia.

Incentive Plus Ltd – www.incentiveplus.co.uk – social, emotional and behavioural resources for children and young people.

Kidpower Family Support Resource, Inc – www.kid-power.org – sensory integration dysfunction section describes this disorder, what behaviour can manifest and how to help.

LDA – www.ldalearning.com – full range of resources for primary school, including extensive handwriting materials, gross and fine motor equipment and materials.

Learning Solutions – www.learning-solutions.co.uk – therapeutic music to enhance development, health and functioning.

National Handwriting Association – www.nha-handwriting.org.uk – a multidisciplinary group based in the United Kingdom. The association promotes the improvement of handwriting standards in schools and supports children with handwriting difficulties. Publications available to EU and non-EU members. Also details of Handwriting Interest Group and membership application forms.

OAASIS – www.oaasis.co.uk – huge range of SEN resources and advice on childhood conditions, including identification, schooling, management.

Pencil Grip – www.thepencilgrip.com – products include a range of pen/pencil grips and other resources including Development by Design toys to encourage skills development through play (www.dbdtoys.com).

PETA UK – www. peta-uk.com – provides a range of photocopiable resources for pre-scissor and scissor skills as well as a range of equipment.

Philip & Tacey – www.philipandtacey.co.uk – resources including angled writing surface and a range of pencil grips.

Posturite – www.posturite.co.uk – includes writing slopes suitable for older children and adults.

ROMPA – www.rompa.com – products, services and concepts for people of all ages with sensory impairments and learning disabilities.

Sensory Integration Network – www.sensoryintegration.org.uk – committed to the promotion and development of sensory integration theory and practice.

Skill Builders Paediatric Occupational Therapy – www.skillbuilders.online.com – includes information on the development of handwriting skills and free downloads of handwriting worksheets and pencil grasp activities.

Southpaw Enterprises – www.southpawenterprises.com – offers sensory integration and developmental products, paediatric therapy equipment, resources and support for therapeutic professionals and health care professionals, schools and families.

SpaceKraft – www.spacekraft.co.uk – develops and manufactures a full range of sensory products for carers and teachers working with special needs children.

SPD (Sensory Processing Disorder Foundation) – www.spdfoundation.net – explains what sensory processing disorder is and links to resources, etc.

Special Direct – www.specialdirect.com – handwriting, fine motor, self-esteem, emotional and allied resources.

Speechmark Publishing Ltd – www.speechmark.net – includes speech and language, emotional development, games and activities.

Taskmaster – www.taskmasteronline.co.uk – for a range of specialist equipment including adapted scissors kit.

TFH Special Needs Toys – www.specialneedstoys.com – a range of products covering physical play, relaxation and daily living activities.

Winslow – www.winslow-cat.com – includes handwriting, self-esteem, special needs.

Professional organisations

BANT (The British Association for Applied Nutrition and Nutritional Therapy), 27 Old Gloucester St, London WC1N 3XX – www.bant.org.uk – professional body for nutritional therapists. Members are qualified in the science of nutrition and provide nutritional therapy.

BABO (British Association of Behavioural Optometrists) – www.babo. co.uk – explains what behavioural optometry is and the role of vision in learning. Includes how to find a behavioural optometrist.

BAOT/COT (British Association/College of Occupational Therapists), College of Occupational Therapists, 106–114 Borough High Street, Southwark, London SE1 1LB – www.cot.org.uk – College of Occupational Therapists Specialist Section – independent practice – www.OTIP.co.uk.

British Chiropractic Association, 59 Castle Street, Reading, Berkshire RG1 7SN – www.chiropractic-uk.co.uk – for advice and assistance with back pain in children (which may be exacerbated by poor sitting positions in class, leaning over flat tables, twisting round in seats to see the teacher, as well as sedentary lifestyle and a lack of opportunity to build up core stability and muscles).

British Dyslexia Association, Unit 8, Bracknell Beeches, Old Bracknell Lane, Bracknell, Berkshire RG12 7BW – www.bdadyslexia.org.uk.

BOA (British Osteopathic Association), 3 Park Terrace, Manor Road, Luton, Bedfordshire LU1 3HN – www.osteopathy.org – a UK professional association of osteopaths.

British Psychological Society, St Andrews House, 48 Princess Road East, Leicester LE1 7DR – www.bps.org.uk – for the Directory of Chartered Psychologists – covers all different specialisms, for example, education.

CSP (Chartered Society of Physiotherapy), 14 Bedford Row, London WC1R 4ED – www.csp.org.uk – the professional, educational and trade union body for chartered physiotherapists.

Christmas Children's Clinic, April Cottage 20 Manor Road, Rusthall, Tunbridge Wells, Kent TN4 8UE – www.christmaschildrensclinic.co.uk – occupational therapists specialising in paediatric assessments and reports.

Dyspraxia Foundation, 8 West Alley, Hitchin, Herts SG5 1EG – www.dyspraxiafoundation.org.uk

Nutrition Science – www.nutritionscience.co.uk – a holistic approach to nutritional therapy, including developmental and autistic spectrum disorders.

INPP (Institute for Neuro-Physiological Psychology), 1 Stanley Street, Chester CH1 2LR – www.inpp.org.uk – (1) a range of excellent publications on the impact of reflexes on childhood and education (2) practitioners and training for a range of developmental issues.

IPSEA (Independent Panel for Special Educational Advice), 6 Carlow Mews, Woodbridge, Suffolk IP12 1EA – including statementing of children with special educational needs – www.ipsea.org.uk

National Autistic Society, 393 City Road, London EC1V 1NG – www.autism.org.uk

RDA (Riding for the Disabled Association), Norfolk House, 1a Tournament Court, Edgehill Drive, Warwick CV34 6LG – www.riding-for-disabled. org.uk – an organisation with a body of volunteers who are dedicated to providing a range of services including riding tuition for children and young people with disabilities.

Royal College of Speech and Language Therapists (England), 2 White Hart Yard, London SE1 1NX – www.rcslt.org – to find a speech and language therapist.

Recommended reading

Ahmad S, Hyde T & Jenkinson J, 2002, *Occupational Therapy Approaches for Secondary Special Needs Practical Classroom Strategies*, Whurr Publishers, London and Philadelphia, PA.

Aquilla P, Sutton S & Yack E, 2007, *Building Bridges through Sensory Integration: Therapy for Children with Autism and Other Pervasive Developmental Disorders*, 2nd edn, Sensory Resources, Las Vegas, NE.

Auer CR & Blumberg SL, 2006, *Parenting a Child with Sensory Processing Disorder: A Family Guide to Understanding and Supporting Your Sensory-Sensitive Child*, New Harbinger, Oakland, CA.

Barsch R, 1995, *Fine Tuning: An Auditory-Visual Training Program*, Academic Therapy Publications, Novato, CA.

Biel L & Peske N (Foreword by Grandin T), 2005, *Raising a Sensory Smart Child: The Definitive Handbook for Helping Your Child with Sensory Integration Issues*, Penguin Group, New York.

Bundy AC, Fisher AG & Murray EA, 1991, *Sensory Integration: Theory and Practice*, F.A. Davis Company, Philadelphia, PA.

Carter R, 1998, *Mapping the Mind*, Phoenix, London.

Case-Smith J (ed), 2001, *Occupational Therapy for Children*, 4th edn, Mosby Inc, St Louis, MO, and London.

Chara KA and Chara PJ Jr with Chara CP, 2004, *Sensory Smarts: A Book for Kids with ADHD or Autism Spectrum Disorders Struggling with Sensory Integration Problems*, Jessica Kingsley Publishers, London.

Goddard S, 1998, *A Teacher's Window into the Child's Mind*, 3rd edn, Fern Ridge Press, Eugene, OR.

Greenfield S, 1997, *The Human Brain: A Guided Tour*, Weidenfeld & Nicolson, London.

Hastings N & Chantrey Wood K, 2002, *Re-organizing Primary Classroom Learning*, Open University Press, Buckingham.

Hannell G, 2003, *Identifying Children with Special Needs: Checklists for Professionals*, SEN Marketing, Wakefield.

Harding J & Meldon-Smith L, 1999, *Helping Young Children to Develop: A Step-by-Step Guide*, Hodder & Stoughton, London.

Harrison K & Scott-Hughes B (eds), 1986, *Look! Look What I Can Do!*, BBC Books, London.

Horowitz LJ & Röst C, 2007, *Helping Hyperactive Kids – A Sensory Integration Approach: Techniques and Tips for Parents and Professionals*, Hunter House Publishers, Alameda, CA.

KBER, 1998, *The Handwriting File*, Kath Balcombe (Educational Resources), Shrewsbury.

Koomar J, Kranowitz C & Szklut S, 2001, *Answers to Questions Teachers Ask about Sensory Integration: Forms, Checklists, and Practical Tools for Teachers and Parents*, Future Horizons, Inc, Arlington, TX.

Kranowitz C, 2005, *The Out-of-sync Child: Recognizing and Coping with Sensory Processing Disorder*, Perigee Book, New York.

Murray-Slutsky C & Paris BA, 2000, *Exploring the Spectrum of Autism and Pervasive Developmental Disorders*, Therapy Skill Builders, Tucson, AR.

Sher B, 1998, *Self-Esteem Games*, John Wiley & Sons Inc, New York.

Sheridan M, 2007, *From Birth to Five Years: Children's Developmental Progress*, 3rd edn, Routledge, Abingdon.

References

Ayres J, 2005, *Sensory Integration and the Child*, Western Psychological Services, Los Angeles, CA.

Centers for Disease Control and Prevention, www.cdc.gov/DiseasesConditions/.

Goddard S, 1998, *A Teacher's Window into the Child's Mind*, 3rd edn, Fern Ridge Press, Eugene, OR.

Hastings N & Chantrey Wood K, 2002, *Re-organizing Primary Classroom Learning*, Open University Press, Buckingham.

Hobbs D & Davidson D, 2000, *Gentle Teaching: A Positive Approach for Challenges of Behavior and Learning*, VHS video, Northern Arizona University, Flagstaff, AZ.

Wing L, 2003, *The Autistic Spectrum: A Guide for Parents and Professionals*, 2nd edn, Robinson Publishing.